Yoga Burns Fat

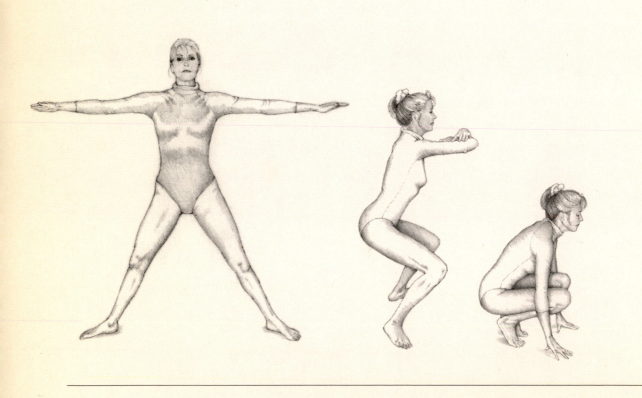

Yoga Burns Fat

Jan Maddern

Fair Winds Press
Gloucester, Massachusetts

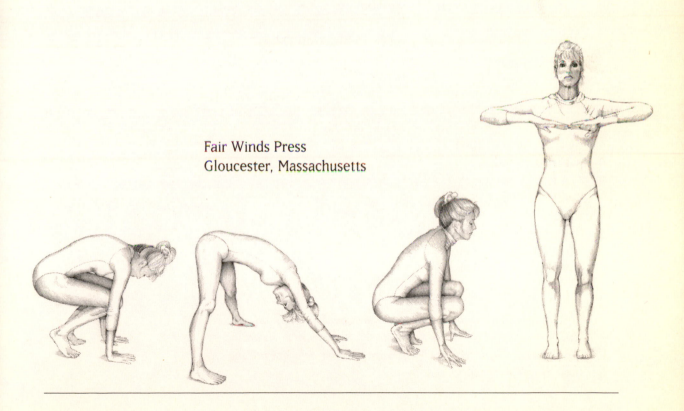

FAIR WINDS

First published in the U.S.A. by
Fair Winds Press
33 Commercial Street
Gloucester, Massachusetts 01930-5089

Library of Congress Cataloging-in-Publication Data
Maddern, Jan.
      Yoga burns fat / Jan Maddern.
            p. cm.
      ISBN 1-931412-66-9
      1. Yoga, Haòtha. 2. Weight loss. I. Title
RA781.7.M335 2002
613.7'046—dc21   2001005954

10 9 8 7 6 5 4 3 2 1

Cover design by Laura Shaw
Cover image by PhotoDisc
Design by Faith Hague
Printed in Canada

*The information in this book is for educational purposes only.
It is not intended to replace the advice of a physician or medical
practitioner. Please see your health care provider before beginning any
new health program.*

Contents

Introduction

We live in a weight-obsessed culture that sets extremely high standards for attractiveness and sets great penalties for being overweight. When it comes to weight loss, many women—overweight or not—believe that their lives would be greatly improved by losing some weight.

Some women would do or pay anything to achieve this goal, hence the lucrative dieting industry and the myriad purveyors of pills, potions, and programs. Clever marketing, aided by the media's endorsement of each new weight-loss miracle, entices millions of people to part with their money for short-term results at best. In a society that craves instant gratification, companies have to keep coming up with products that promise quicker, more fabulous results.

Yet we know that statistically, most people who lose weight end up gaining it back. Each new product or claim—which often contradicts previous ones—serves only to confuse the average weight-loss consumer. People end up not knowing what to believe, eat, or use. And so the problem persists worldwide: in westernized and industrialized countries, people are getting heavier, despite the increasing availability of health clubs, weight-loss clinics, and low-fat foods. Obesity is now recognized as a chronic, life-threatening disease.

Why Yoga?

The practice of hatha yoga has been proven throughout the ages to be one of the most effective ways to create and maintain a healthy lifestyle that, over time, will lead to a permanent, healthy weight. *Hatha yoga* is the science of the physical body, which includes a range of styles from gentle to athletic. The practice of hatha yoga includes postures (*asanas*); breathing techniques (*pranayama*); and visualization, relaxation, and meditation techniques.

When you look at the bodies of regular yoga practitioners, you see long, lean muscles and strong, toned bodies.

Yoga poses stretch and tone the entire range of muscles and increase the total percentage of lean muscle tissue in the body. This process gives muscles definition and increases the body's overall metabolic rate for burning fat. The combination of increased body heat and deep breathing rapidly releases toxins through the skin and the breath.

Benefits of This Program

Several yoga poses, combined in a sequence and performed dynamically, are called a *vinyasa*. They greatly enhance the way your body burns fat by increasing body heat and thus raising your metabolic rate.

This book contains seven routines to help you attain a healthy weight. Each yoga routine contains stretches, a vinyasa, postural exercises, a breathing technique, and a visualization technique. From the moment you first practice these techniques, you will notice benefits. You will move more easily and have better concentration and balance; you also will feel more energized, determined, self-confident, relaxed, and inwardly calm.

You can safely reach your desired weight-loss goals by using these yoga routines. Day by day, you will increase the aerobic capacity of your heart; your body's ability to burn fat; and your physical, mental, and emotional stamina. By regularly practicing these techniques and eating a balanced diet, you can attain and maintain a permanent, healthy weight without pills, programs, or payments. You can confidently expect to drop a dress size in 7 weeks.

Through the regular practice of yoga, you also can avoid many of the health problems associated with being overweight, such as

- ➤ stress on the heart;
- ➤ diabetes;
- ➤ high blood pressure and cholesterol levels, which can increase risk of heart disease;
- ➤ arthritis and pressure on the joints;
- ➤ risk of sleep disorders such as sleep apnea, which is associated with heart disease;
- ➤ risk of gallstones;

➤ hormone imbalances, which can increase the risk of breast or endometrial cancer and menstrual irregularities; and

➤ premature death.

This book shares with you the secrets of yogic weight loss and maintenance that have been passed down through the ages. By practicing the yoga routines presented in this book regularly, you will not only look more healthy. You also will maintain steady energy and sugar levels throughout the day, avoiding unhealthy cravings; improve digestive and eliminatory function for the effective use of the food you eat and elimination of waste; speed up your metabolic rate to burn fat, so you don't lose just water weight; create a healthy self-image of the person you would like to be; and finally, stick to a weight-loss program without becoming depressed. In total, you will *feel* healthy because you will *be* healthy.

How to Use This Book

The information presented in this book can be used alone or in conjunction with any other weight-loss program. The initial program runs for 7 weeks to improve your body's ability to lose weight safely and efficiently. Each day's 30-minute routine contains six simple steps, and the seven routines are progressively more challenging.

Although the program time line assumes that you will master a new routine every week, proceed more slowly if you need to; every body is different and presents different limitations. If you already exercise regularly and are moderately fit, you probably can safely practice these vinyasa sequences, one vinyasa a day, each routine for a week. However, if you are just starting an exercise program, practice each routine at your own pace. Do not move on to the next routine until you feel comfortable in the current one. If you progress within your own limitations, you can confidently expect to improve the way your body burns fat over time.

A New Way of Life

Diets are not miracle cures; in fact, the original meaning of the word *diet* is "way of life." Practiced regularly in conjunction with eating a healthy balanced diet, hatha yoga offers you a safe route to the weight that is right for you. The more regularly you practice and the more you moderate your eating patterns, the more effective and permanent your weight loss will be.

By choosing yoga as an approach to weight loss, you can get off the diet industry treadmill that drains your energy as well as your purse. Leave yo-yo dieting behind forever as you develop a healthy, balanced approach to permanent weight loss. Working from the inside out, you can restore the balance in your body systems and glands that control your metabolic rate, appetite, moods, and sleep patterns.

The routines presented in this book help you reach your target weight efficiently and will change the way you feel about your body shape and image, laying the basis for a healthier, happier, and more meaningful lifestyle. You then can trust your body's inner wisdom to take care of the physical so that you can focus on higher mental, emotional, and spiritual aspirations. As you regain control of your life, expect to see positive changes—and enjoy the new you!

Warning: *The information presented in this book is of a general nature. Being overweight can cause serious health problems, which in its worst form— extreme obesity—can even cause premature death. This book is not intended to replace the services of a trained health-care practitioner, who can consult with you about matters related to your own health or symptoms that require diagnosis and immediate treatment. If you have high blood pressure, diabetes, or other weight-related health problems, consult your medical practitioner before beginning this program.*

chapter one

Beyond Dieting: The Yoga Approach

The benefits of the yoga routines presented in this book go far beyond those of conventional diet plans, which usually suggest eliminating certain food groups and throwing yourself into a frantic exercise routine to lose weight quickly. The yoga approach is far more effective in helping you reach and maintain a healthy weight. It also is more enjoyable and easier (both physically and psychologically) than rigid eating or exercise programs.

When you practice the yoga routines regularly, you do not need to obsess about how many hours you exercise each week. The practice of yoga teaches you to listen to your intuitive self. You will know how much or how little to practice each day, according to your body's needs. From the moment you practice your first routine, you will notice benefits. You will move more easily; have improved balance; be able to concentrate better; and feel more energized, determined, and self-confident yet relaxed and inwardly calm. The more you enjoy your practice, the more you will want to practice. In this way, yoga

Did You Know?

Although vegetarianism is preferred by many yoga practitioners worldwide, you do not have to be vegetarian to enjoy the benefits of yoga. You also do not have to give up sweets, alcohol, or sex. You start from where you are and let yoga work its magic from within!

A common-sense approach to nutrition will help you build a healthy lifestyle. Choose foods from all food groups if you wish, so that you are nourished by all the nutrients that you need to reach and maintain a healthy weight. Fresh fruits and vegetables form the basis of a sensible diet; eat five to seven servings each day. (A soup and salad a day keep the weight at bay!) High-fiber foods will make you feel full with smaller portions. And plain, pure water is essential for nourishing all the cells of the body; drink at least eight glasses of water every day.

becomes a self-regulating tool for optimum health. The benefits accrue from week to week, and the better you feel about yourself, the more you will want to take care of yourself. You will adopt increasingly healthier behaviors as your moods, appetite, and sleep patterns are bought back into balance. You will consciously choose healthy, nutritious foods; drink an abundance of water; exercise daily; and feel more relaxed and nourished overall. Weight loss will follow naturally.

Why "Working from Within" is Better Than "Working Out"

The practice of hatha yoga develops an awareness of working from within to enhance your well-being rather than striving for some external, idealized image of yourself. Because yoga is not competitive, your ego and any aggressive feelings can take a backseat while practicing, so that your mind can become quiet. A quiet mind allows you to reflect and become aware of what is happening in your body.

Working from within, you get to know your body and what it is capable of performing. In this way, you learn not to overextend or damage muscles and joints. You can simply "be" in a pose or move into the flow of a sequence without distraction, while consciously stretching and breathing and reflecting on your self-image. This quiet, reflective time allows you to access all those motivational and inspirational thoughts deep in your subconscious mind.

By consciously directing the vitality or life force (called *prana*) that comes from deep breathing into your mental images of a healthy body, you can effectively energize your thoughts. By creating a clear mental image of your body returning to a healthy optimum weight, you activate your body's own intuitive healing system. It will restore balance to the workings of all the glands that control your weight and appetite. This method has a far more beneficial effect on the body–mind–emotions connection than working out purely to burn fat.

The yoga routines presented in this book convey two major benefits:

➤ They increase circulation to the major digestive organs to improve their function, so that constipation, water retention, and bloating are eliminated.

➤ They improve the supply of fresh oxygenated blood to the major endocrine glands that control your appetite, moods, and sleep patterns.

The glands, which help to regulate your weight, include

➤ thyroid gland, which controls oxygen and energy levels in the body and, hence, your metabolic rate;

➤ pancreas, which controls sugar and energy levels throughout the day to avoid sugar highs and lows;

➤ adrenal glands, which control stress levels to reduce fears, self-doubts, and anxiety, all of which can hinder a weight-loss program;

➤ thymus gland, which controls the immune system;

➤ parathyroid gland, which controls sleep patterns; and

➤ pineal and pituitary glands, which control moods and appetite.

More Than Just Weight Loss

You may have picked up this book because you want to lose a dress size. Yet the practice of hatha yoga offers you the opportunity to go beyond that, to achieve a healthy weight and maintain it forever. In addition to improving the aerobic capacity of your heart and increasing your metabolic rate to burn fat, you will learn how to

➤ visualize something you want in your life so clearly and consistently that your mind is open to positive suggestions about how to achieve that goal, whether it is losing weight, getting a new job, or having a more satisfying relationship;

➤ use your breath to calm your emotions and mind so that you can manage any fears, doubts, or anxieties that are stopping you from reaching your goals;

➤ like and value yourself the way you are, and to be thankful for all that you have achieved already in your life; and

➤ make conscious decisions about your lifestyle, based on common-sense nutritional guidelines plus your intuition, which will allow you to maintain a healthy weight.

When you practice the techniques presented in this book, you will join millions of people who have experienced the profound benefits of practicing yoga regularly. An increasing number of film stars and athletes do yoga, and 15 million Americans include some form of yoga in their fitness routine—twice as many as did 5 years ago. Seventy-five percent of all health clubs in the United States now offer yoga classes, for people just like yourself.

The physical benefits of returning to a healthy weight are enough to prevent obesity-related illnesses. Yet it is the emotional, mental, and spiritual nurturing of the practice that often brings people to yoga. Once you try it, your cravings for food, alcohol, and other stimulants may be replaced with a healthy craving: living life to the fullest!

chapter two

The Power of Vinyasas

Yoga poses, or asanas, stretch and tone the muscles, massage the internal organs, tone the nerves, and regulate the body's hormonal output—all of which improves overall well-being. Each asana brings certain benefits individually. But when several asanas are combined into a flowing sequence (a vinyasa), their value is enhanced by the combination of the poses as well as the speed at which they are practiced.

This book contains seven yoga routines. They progress from easier to more difficult, so you continue to be challenged as your strength and flexibility improve. Each routine is presented in six sections:

➤ STRETCH AND TONE, a gentle warm-up for your muscles;
➤ IMPROVE POSTURE, an exercise to tone your abdominal muscles;
➤ IMPROVE DIGESTION AND ELIMINATION, a *bandha* (a strong abdominal exercise that massages all the internal organs to improve their function) that helps prevent water retention, bloating, and constipation;
➤ IMPROVE METABOLIC RATE, a vinyasa to boost your metabolic rate;
➤ BREATHE, a technique to increase your metabolic rate and focus your mind; and
➤ VISUALIZE, a guide to increasing positive thinking.

Did You Know?

Most women gain an average of about 18 pounds (8 kilograms) of body fat between the ages of 20 and 50. According to Donna Aston, author of *Fat or Fiction— Are You Living a Fairytale?* (Hybrid Publishers, Australia, 1999), unbelievably, it takes an excess of only 5–10 calories a day (overeaten or not burned) for this weight gain to occur. Conversely, only 5–10 calories saved or burned off each day can prevent this weight gain.

Potential Benefits

Seven yoga routines have been designed especially for this book. If you follow the instructions carefully, practice regularly, and eat a healthy, balanced diet, you can confidently expect to drop a dress size by the end of the 7 weeks.

The routines convey several benefits:

➤ **Warm-up stretches** prepare your body for more vigorous exercise and help avoid injury.

➤ **Posture-improving exercises** improve the tone and strength of your abdominal and back muscles, so you will look and feel slimmer.

➤ **Bandhas** improve the muscle tone of your digestive and eliminatory system as well as improve the health and function of your pancreas, which controls sugar levels.

➤ **Vinyasas** improve the way your body loses and maintains weight by nourishing your endocrine glands, which control weight, and by increasing the aerobic capacity of your heart.

➤ **Breathing techniques** increase your oxygen levels and your metabolic rate so your body can process food more efficiently.

➤ **Visualizations** help you to release any negative attitudes, beliefs, or values that might be sapping your energy and preventing you from reaching your goals. They improve your overall self-image through learning to value attributes other than a size-10 body! They train your mind to picture something clearly, consistently, and long enough so that you can attain your desired goals.

As you practice these dynamic sequences regularly, you will increase the percentage of strong, lean muscle tissue in your body. Each vinyasa builds strength, tone, and flexibility in all of the muscles, joints, and ligaments of the body as well as bone strength, because the vinyasas are weight-bearing exercises. Studies by Miriam Nelson, a researcher at Tufts University and author of *Strong Women Stay Young* (Bantam Doubleday Dell, 2000), says that increasing muscle mass not only promotes aerobic activity, which burns calories, but also boosts your metabolic rate.

When muscles grow, the body produces more beneficial enzymes, which can help the muscles store and use fuel and aid in waste disposal. Muscle-building vinyasas, combined with common-sense nutrition, are very effective in helping you reach a healthy weight, gradually and permanently, by increasing your metabolic rate.

When you breathe deeply while practicing the vinyasas in each routine, you increase the oxygenated blood supply to the muscles of your body, which raises your metabolic rate. With each breath, your body cleanses itself with oxygen-saturated blood. The toxins are then naturally discarded from your body through perspiration, exhalation, and elimination. This explains why you might feel hot and sweaty, a bit out of breath, and suddenly feel the need to use the bathroom while working through these sequences!

By the end of 7 weeks, you can confidently expect to look and feel more positive about yourself and your body image. Scales are not a good measurement of success, so do not weigh yourself during the 7 weeks; you will be building muscle tissue to make you leaner and more toned, and muscle weighs more than fat. You will know from the way you look and feel that you are making progress.

How to Use the Routines

Seven routines are presented in this book, and each routine takes approximately 30 minutes to complete. If you cannot find 30 minutes a day to work on improving your health and well-being, then you might ask yourself, "Who is controlling my life?" Certainly not you! You are probably putting the needs of everyone else before your own.

The secret of yoga is that as your self-esteem, self-motivation, and self-respect improve, so will your ability to value your own needs as much as those of others. To achieve and maintain a healthy weight while enjoying countless physical and emotional benefits, follow a few simple guidelines:

➤ Begin by reading The Power of Vinyasas (Chapter 2) and The Power of Visualization (Chapter 3).
➤ Practice the Warm-Up stretches (beginning on page 19) until you are familiar with them. Always warm up before practicing a routine.
➤ Practice Routine 1 every day for one week. Initially, allow yourself extra time to learn the routine.

- Start the first repetition in each vinyasa slowly, and increase your speed toward the last repetition, so that you build up heat in your body and start to sweat.
- The second week, if you feel comfortable practicing Routine 1, practice Routine 2 every day.
- Work your way through the seven routines, practicing a routine a day, for a week or longer (until you feel comfortable with the entire routine), until you have completed the seven routines. Do not move on to the next routine until you have mastered the current one.
- Practice the most strenuous routines when you are most energized.
- Eat a healthy, balanced diet.
- After the initial 7-week program, alternate and mix elements from different routines to avoid boredom.

The more you practice these routines, the more you will come to appreciate that losing and maintaining weight is a holistic affair. There are no shortcuts, and it requires total awareness of mind, body, and emotions to be successful.

Instructions for Practicing

The vinyasas need to be approached with care, because when they are done dynamically, they are quite strenuous.

- If you are moderately fit or mildly overweight, you can practice the routines safely in the comfort of your own home. If you are very overweight, consult your medical practitioner first, then work with an experienced yoga teacher before you embark on this program.
- Consult your medical practitioner if you have back, neck, or joint problems; high blood pressure; diabetes; or asthma.
- Do not eat for an hour before practicing; even then, eat only something light, such as some fresh fruit or yogurt.
- Establish a regular time of day to practice. Warm up first, then spend about 30 minutes practicing one routine at a time, for a week at a time. It is important to complete an entire routine—stretching, posture-improving exercise, vinyasa, breathing technique, and visualization—for maximum effect.

- Practice on a floor surface that is not slippery or use a nonskid mat (called a "sticky mat," available at sports stores and from yoga suppliers).
- Practice in bare feet, and wear loose, comfortable clothing. Do not practice in air conditioning if possible. (These routines will build heat in your body, and air conditioning can cause a chill when your body is still again.)
- Use an aromatherapy diffuser or burn incense while you practice. For an uplifting effect, use scents such as bergamot, geranium, orange, rosewood, sandalwood, or ylang ylang. To clear your mind, try using eucalyptus, pine, or tea tree.
- Listen to your favorite nonintrusive music while you practice.
- After completing the vinyasa, cover yourself with a large towel or blanket to complete the breathing and visualization work, which requires you to sit still.
- Drink a glass of water after practicing to help eliminate toxins from your body.

Warm-Up

The following warm-up stretches lubricate stiff joints, increase circulation, and improve your flexibility. They will make your practice of the routines more comfortable and help you avoid injury. Use your visualization skills with each stretch to improve their benefits.

Visualize yourself moving intuitively into and out of the stretch according to your body's needs. Be aware that rushing too quickly into an exercise program is a sure-fire route to lower-back pain, so be patient with yourself. However, carrying a little extra weight is not a limitation; often a person with a large build can be both stronger and more flexible than a person who has been working out. For example, repetitive choreographed routines can lead to the overuse of muscle groups and joints as well as shortening and tightening of the muscles, leading to inflexibility and muscle fatigue.

Spine Stretch

Benefits

Stretches the spine; tones the hamstrings and muscles of the shoulders, neck, and spine

Focus

When bringing your weight back onto your heels, visualize a strong upside-down "V" shape. Actively stretch through your arms and legs as you lift your hips to the ceiling.

1. Stand with your feet hip-width apart and your arms extended to the sides at shoulder height, palms facing down.
2. Bend forward. Place your palms flat on the floor (bend your knees if necessary), and "walk" your hands about 4 feet away from your feet.
3. Lift your hips up and back, so that your weight comes back firmly onto your heels, which stretch toward the floor. Extend your arms strongly; your spine should be slightly arched. Drop your head down between your arms, and push your chest toward the tops of your thighs.
4. Shift your weight forward onto your palms and then back strongly to shift your weight onto your heels again. Repeat this back-and-forth motion 7 times.
5. "Walk" your hands back toward your legs, step your legs 4–6 feet apart, bend your arms, and grab your elbows with your opposite hands.
6. Let your upper body hang forward from your hips, bringing your elbows and head toward to the floor. Breathe deeply, and feel your spine extend.
7. Slowly come up to a standing position with a straight back and hands still clasped around your elbows. Release your hands to your sides, and shrug your shoulders.

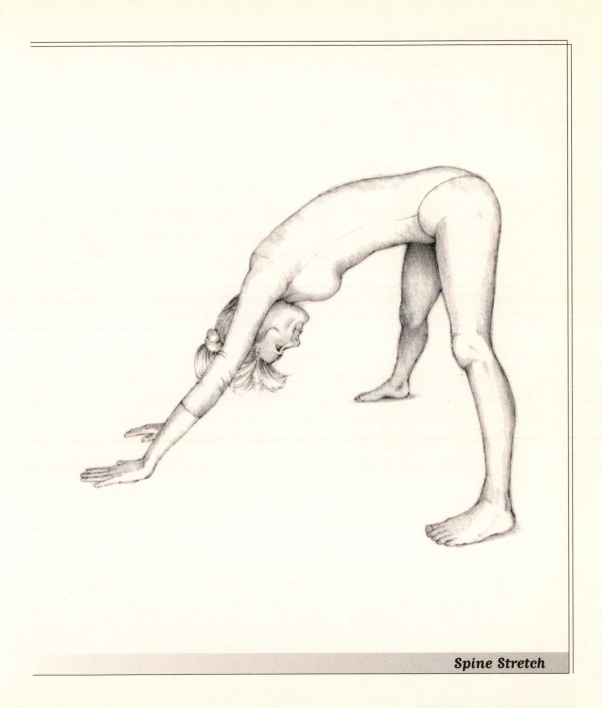

Spine Stretch

Shoulder Swings

Benefits

Opens up the shoulders, hips, and neck to release stiffness; improves range of movement in the joints

Focus

Rotate your head as far as possible to each side to improve the flexibility of your neck. Keep your legs strong and kneecaps locked for balance.

1. Stand upright with your legs 4–6 feet apart. Inhaling, circle your arms wide and up over your head; exhaling, bend forward. Place your palms flat on the floor in front of you (bend your knees if necessary), shoulder-width apart.

2. Inhaling, look to the right and swing your right arm in a wide circle to the right as far as possible, pulling your right shoulder and right hip back. Exhaling, place your right palm flat on the floor in front of you.

3. Inhaling, look to the left and swing your left arm in a wide circle to the left as far as possible, pulling your left shoulder and left hip back. Exhaling, place your left palm flat on the floor in front of you.

4. Repeat this swinging movement 7 times to each side, inhaling on the stretch and exhaling on the return to the center in steady, even breaths.

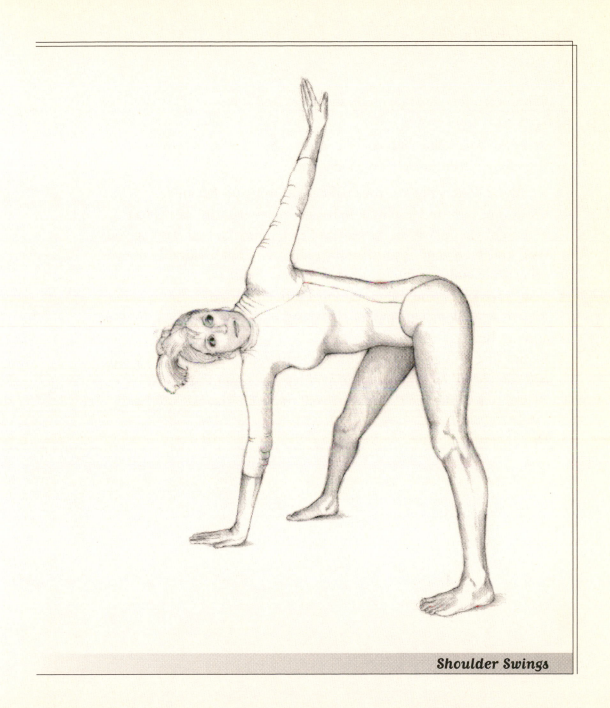

Shoulder Swings

Spinal Rolls

Benefits

Releases tension along the neck, shoulders, and spine

Focus

Roll onto your spine with control, vertebra by vertebra, so you activate your abdominal muscles at the same time.

1. Sit on the floor, and cross your right ankle over your left ankle.
2. Clasp your toes, and lean back to balance on your sitting bones (the bottom of your pelvis, in the center of each buttock). Still clasping your toes, straighten your legs toward the ceiling, and roll backward onto your spine while pulling your feet up, toward your head.
3. Bend your knees, and roll forward to a sitting position.
4. Repeat the slow rocking motion, backward onto your spine and forward again, 7 times.
5. Return to a sitting position. Cross your left ankle over your right ankle, and complete 7 backward-and-forward repetitions on this side.
6. Return to a sitting position, release your toes, and uncross your legs.

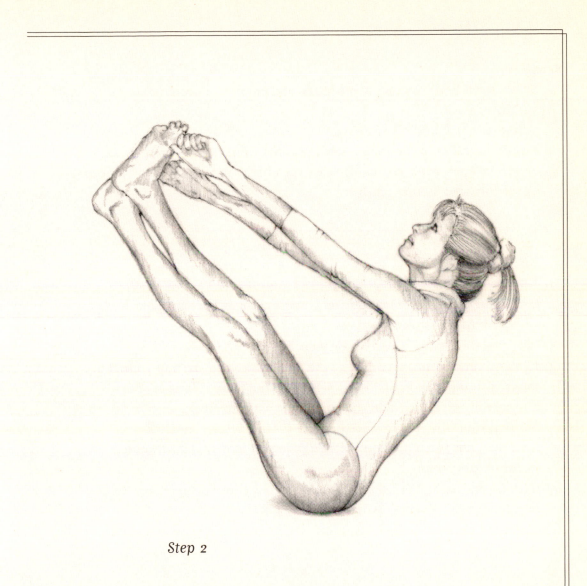

Step 2

Child's Pose

Benefits

Slows down heart rate, body processes, and emotions; promotes looking within

(**Note:** Use Child's Pose after any stretch or after a vinyasa to quiet and focus your mind, promoting a sense of inner stillness. This stretch keeps your hips open while resting between yoga poses and allows your spine and upper thighs to stretch gently.)

Focus

Bring your buttocks as close to the floor as possible. Widen your feet and knees if necessary.

1. Kneel on the floor; lean back, and place your hands on your calves.
2. Grab your calves, roll them outward, and sit deeply between your heels; let your buttocks sink toward the floor.
3. Let your arms hang, hands beside your hips, palms facing back.
4. Keeping your buttocks as close to the floor as possible, stretch your chin forward, and gently lower your forehead to the floor. (**Note:** If your buttocks lift up rather than stay in contact with the floor, concentrate on pushing your buttocks toward the floor to stretch your spine. If your head does not reach the floor, place a pillow or folded blanket under your forehead for comfort.)
5. Round your back, and let your shoulders drop closer to the floor. Relax into the pose in a very passive way. Breathe deeply.

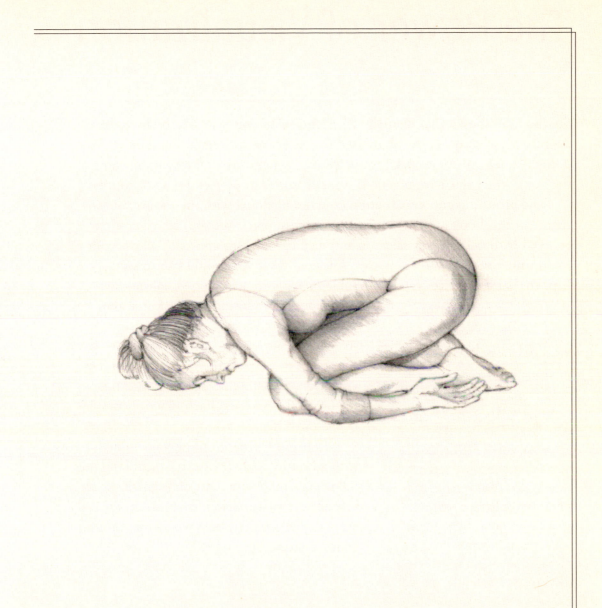

Child's Pose

chapter three

The Power of Visualization

Studies have shown that mentally rehearsing what you want the body to do stimulates pathways in the brain used for the actual movements and, in so doing, "tunes up" the muscles for maximum benefit. Mental rehearsal is nothing new—the yogis have practiced it for centuries to perfect a pose or routine.

The breathing and visualization exercises included with each routine presented in this book are practiced with slowness, precision, and concentration coupled with periods of relaxation and meditation. This approach allows your mind time to formulate a very clear image of what you would like to see happen. With practice, you will be able to apply these strong visualization skills not only to losing weight but also to achieving other lifestyle goals. To ensure success in your weight loss program, it is as important to practice the breathing and visualization techniques as it is to practice the physical workouts. Each practice complements the other.

To begin reprogramming your mind with a healthy body image, try practicing the following simple visualization exercise. Practice the visualization for 15 minutes every day in a quiet place, whenever you find yourself sitting or lying still.

Did You Know?

Most people fail to lose weight and keep it off not because they lack willpower or self-discipline but because they lack the visualization skills that are needed to program the subconscious mind.

The subconscious mind can be reached only through visualization because it "thinks" in pictures, not words. In our fast-paced world, in which we expect results instantly, our only mistake is to think so quickly that the picture does not have time to make a lasting imprint on the subconscious.

Cross-Legged Position

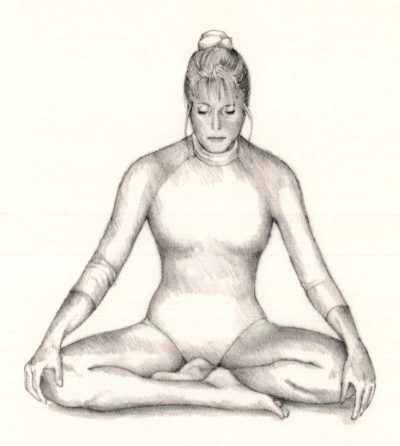

➤ Place a cushion on the floor, and sit on it in Cross-Legged Position. (**Note:** If this position is not comfortable, sit on a folded towel to tilt your hips forward and take the pressure off your knees. Alternatively, sit with your legs stretched out in front, leaning against a wall if necessary, or sit in a chair.) Rest your hands on your knees, palms facing up or down.

➤ Close your eyes, and be perfectly still; you cannot relax completely unless your body is perfectly still.

- Inhale deeply and slowly, then exhale with a gentle sigh.
- Let your breath come and go in an easy, unhurried way, paying attention to the rise and fall of your chest with each breath. (**Note:** Do not force your breath into any pattern; observe it as if you were outside your body.)
- With each exhalation, let all the weight of your body sink down into your buttocks. With each inhalation, feel as if you are being pulled up by a string attached to the crown of your head while the base of your spine is anchored to the floor.
- Let your logical thinking (all that planning about what you are going to do next) subside, and silence the chatter in your mind so that your mind can rest. Do not try to stop the thoughts; watch them come and go. The more detached you become, the more your mind will become quiet. Observe all that is going on in your body and mind.
- Let the "observer" go, but let the "observing" continue.
- Be as still as a statue. Watch your mind become quiet, and visualize your life as you would like to be—the way you would like to look, speak, and interact with people; the sort of relationship you would like to have with a partner; the career path or hobbies that you would like to have. Continue the visualization for a few minutes. (**Note:** If you cannot "see" this image clearly, then for the moment, just think about it. The vision will come with practice.)
- In the silence, refine this image of yourself as you would like to be for 10–15 minutes, until it is very clear in your mind.
- To finish the exercise, gently begin to deepen your breath. (You may have noticed throughout the visualization that as you became more relaxed, you almost forgot to breathe.)
- Stretch your arms out in front of you, then overhead.

➤ Rub your palms together until your hands are very warm, then place them over your eyes.

➤ Release your palms, blink, stand up, and stretch your body to each side to awaken your spine.

You will feel relaxed and alert, ready to get on with your day, knowing that you have imprinted a very clear image of your ideal self on your mind. Your subconscious will be open and receptive to the suggestions that will make this vision a reality. The more you practice, the more effective the results will be, so keep on refining the image of yourself as you would like to be until it is very clear in your mind. Expect this vision to become a reality sooner than you think!

chapter four

Routine 1

Each of the vinyasas in this book is designed to increase your percentage of lean muscle over time. Gaining 1 pound of lean muscle is enough to burn approximately 25 calories a day and can prevent weight gain as you age. You can easily gain lean muscle tissue by consistently increasing the amount of time spent on any physical exercise: gardening, housework, walking, or sporting activities. It does not have to be formal exercise; just keep moving, because it all adds up at the end of the day. Practiced dynamically and regularly in combination with your other daily activities, vinyasas will keep you lean and toned, and your resulting high metabolic rate will burn excess calories. (Unfortunately, it works both ways; for every pound of lean muscle tissue you lose, either due to inactivity or lack of essential nutrients, you will burn approximately 25 calories less each day.)

Routine 1 introduces you to one of the best-loved vinyasas, Salute to the Sun, which quickly stretches and tones all the muscles and improves the function of the hormonal system, which controls mood and appetite. The poses convey several benefits:

Did You Know?

When you make time to quiet your mind and listen to the silence within, you will find all the answers for being a fulfilled, happy human being. You need only create the right conditions to hear this wisdom by regularly quieting your mind.

➤ **Head-to-Knee Stretch** releases tension throughout your spine and the backs of your hamstrings, allowing you to extend in Salute to the Sun.
➤ **Pelvic Rocking** makes you aware of the way that subtle stretches can improve the strength and tone of your abdominal and back muscles.
➤ **Stomach Bandha** tightens abdominal muscles and improves the way that food is moved through your eliminatory system.

It also massages your pancreas, so that you have a steady flow of energy throughout the day, to avoid sugar cravings.

➤ **Vinyasa 1**, Salute to the Sun, improves the flexibility of your spine and major joints and speeds up your breathing rate and heart rate to increase your metabolic rate.

➤ **Present-Minded Awareness Breath** keeps you focused in the present moment as you coordinate your breath with leg and arm movements.

➤ **Creating a Healthy Self-Image** is a visualization that helps you release old thought patterns and ideas (e.g., feelings of sadness, hurt, resentment, or guilt over the past or present) that may be preventing you from reaching your goals by taking up your best energies.

STRETCH AND TONE

Head-to-Knee Stretch

Benefits

Increases blood flow to the brain; lowers blood pressure; promotes inner stillness

Focus

Lengthen your spine on the inhalation with your chin extended, then soften your spine on the exhalation. Let your head and neck hang freely; do not strain.

1. Stand with your legs 4–6 feet apart, arms outstretched at shoulder height.

2. Exhaling, bend forward. Place your palms flat on the floor between your feet (bend your knees if necessary).

3. Turn your right foot out to the side a little; "walk" your hands over to your right foot, and place them on either side of your right ankle or on top of your right foot.

4. Inhaling, lengthen through the spine. Exhaling, soften the body and extend through the chin rather than trying to put the head on the knee. Continue lengthening and extending the spine as you breathe deeply 7 times.

5. Exhaling, "walk" your hands back to the front.

6. Inhaling, come up to a standing position.

7. Turn your right foot to the front and your left foot out to the side. Repeat the stretch on your left side for 7 breaths.

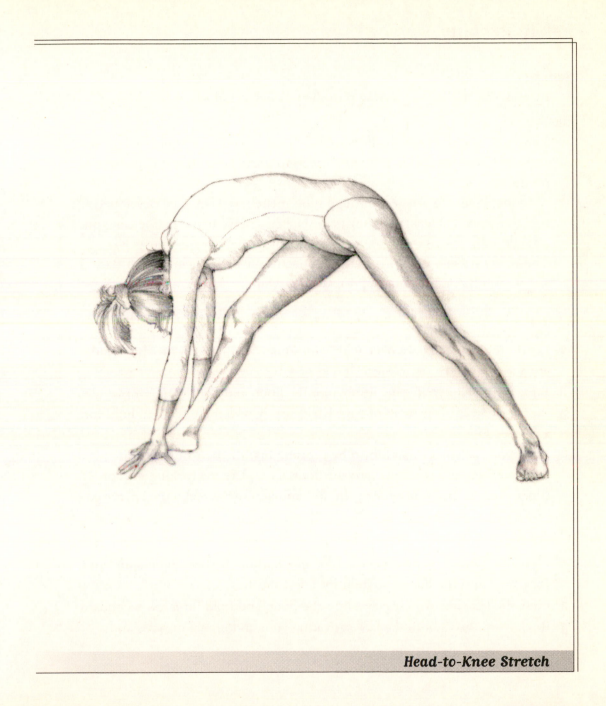

Head-to-Knee Stretch

IMPROVE POSTURE

Pelvic Rocking

Benefits

Increases flexibility for moving into the poses that follow

Focus

Press each vertebra into the floor, one by one, as you rock your pelvis. Use your abdominal muscles, not your knees, to move your weight between points.

(**Note:** These "awareness through movement" exercises were developed by Dr. Moshe Feldenkrais. They help the body move better by focusing on a single subject—in this case, making tiny movements with your pelvis. These movements are subtle but very effective in strengthening your back and abdominal muscles to improve your posture.)

STAGE 1

1. Lie on the floor on your back with your knees bent, feet on the floor, and arms at your sides. Your knees should be a comfortable distance apart.
2. Press the base of your spine firmly into the floor, and hold for a few seconds.
3. Press your waist (the small of your back) firmly into the floor, and hold for a few seconds.
4. Rock your pelvis back and forth by pressing first the base of your spine, then the back of your waist into the floor. Complete the rocking motion 10 times, then relax. Notice how your abdominal muscles feel more energized.

STAGE 2

1. Press the right side of your pelvis (the area midway between your spine and your hip) into the floor, and hold for a few seconds.
2. Press the left side of your pelvis into the floor, and hold for a few seconds.
3. Rock from the right to the left, activating your abdominal muscles and

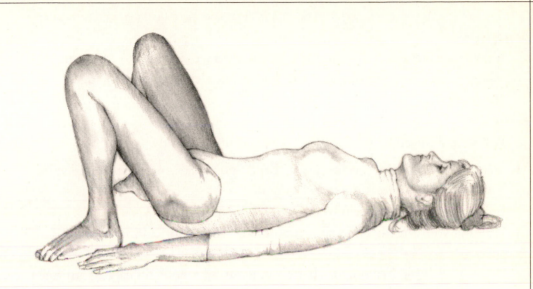

keeping your knees still. (**Note:** Keep your buttocks on the floor throughout the exercise.) Complete the rocking motion 10 times, then relax.

STAGE 3

1. Imagine drawing a circle among four points focused on in Stages 1 and 2.
2. Begin in a counterclockwise direction by pressing the back of your waist into the floor. Next, press the left side of your pelvis, the base of your spine, the right side of your pelvis, and the back of your waist again. (This is one rotation.) Complete 10 rotations, as slowly as possible, making the movement among the four points as broad a circle as possible.
3. Change to a clockwise direction. Press the back of your waist into the floor. Next, press the right side of your pelvis, the base of your spine, the left side of your pelvis, and the back of your waist again. Complete 10 rotations.
4. Hug your knees to your chest, and rock backward and forward.

Pelvic Rocking

IMPROVE DIGESTION AND ELIMINATION

Stomach Bandha

Adapted from Lucille Wood, Gita International Yoga Australia, with permission.

Benefits

Improves function of the pancreas, which produces insulin, to maintain steady energy levels throughout the day and moderate unhealthy sugar cravings

Focus

Pull your abdominal muscles back, up, and under tightly.

1. Stand with your legs 4–6 feet apart. Bend your knees and squat; place your hands on your knees, fingertips facing in.
2. Inhale, then exhale forcefully through an open mouth.
3. Holding your breath, close your mouth, and tuck your chin into your chest.
4. Suck your abdominal muscles back, up, and under your rib cage. Continue to hold your breath for a count of 7.
5. Release your abdominal muscles.
6. Inhaling, straighten your legs and come up. Exhaling, bend forward and hang loosely.
7. Repeat the sequence 3 more times. Practice to gradually increase to 7 repetitions.

(**Note:** If you are not used to holding your breath, this exercise may make you cough or feel a little dizzy at first. If it does, exhale and release your head down between your legs, then try again.)

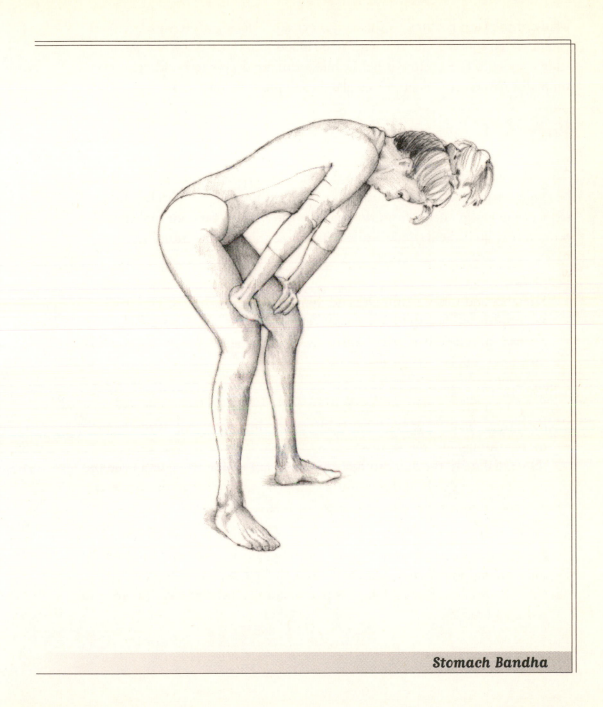

Stomach Bandha

IMPROVE METABOLIC RATE

Many of the yoga postures in this vinyasa create a "lock" or pressure over a gland, which squeezes out the stale, toxic blood from your body like water from a sponge. The posture is held while breathing deeply to build up a fresh supply of oxygenated blood to the gland to improve its function.

Vinyasa 1

The most popular vinyasa, Salute to the Sun, is a 12-step sequence. You should be able to complete seven repetitions in 10–15 minutes. Symbolically, this sequence draws in energy from the sun so it can be used for your highest purposes throughout the day; ideally, it is done first thing in the morning.

Benefits
Stretches and tones all muscles and joints; strengthens bones; improves respiratory and heart rates; increases energy level; improves concentration, cleanses the glandular system of toxins; lifts depression and anxiety; speeds metabolic rate for weight maintenance

Focus
Keep your movements smooth and graceful; keep your breathing even and rhythmic. Envision yourself being inwardly calm and serene as you breathe deeply throughout the sequence.
(**Note:** Salute to the Sun can be practiced as fast as you like—at an aerobic pace, or more slowly and mindfully. However you choose to practice this vinyasa, complete the warm-up stretches first.)

1. Stand with your feet hip-width apart and your hands in front of your chest, palms together, fingers pointing up. Inhaling, circle your arms wide out to the side, and join your palms overhead. Exhaling, return your hands to your chest, palms together, fingers pointing up. Slowly release your arms to rest at your sides.

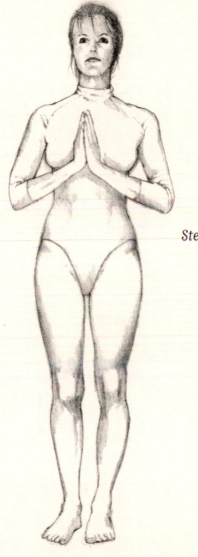

Step 1

Vinyasa 1

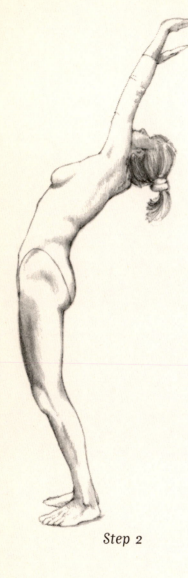

2. Inhaling, extend your arms overhead, and arch backward slightly. (Note: This pose creates a lock over your parathyroid glands, for calcium balance, and your adrenal glands, which control stress levels.)

3. Exhaling, bend forward, keeping your back straight. Place your palms flat on the floor, outside your feet (bend your knees if necessary). Tuck your chin under. (**Note:** This pose creates a lock over your thyroid gland, which balances your metabolic rate.)

Step 2

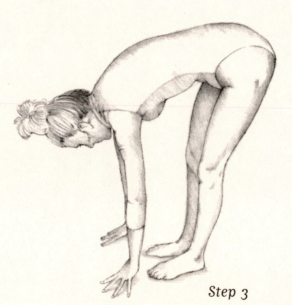

Step 3

4. Inhaling, step your left leg straight back. Bend your right knee in a forward lunge. Extend through your chin. (**Note:** This pose massages your internal organs in your abdomen to encourage elimination.)

5. Exhaling, extend your right leg straight back and tighten your abdominal muscles while supporting your body weight on locked arms and your toes. (**Note:** This weight-bearing pose tones your arm and leg muscles.)

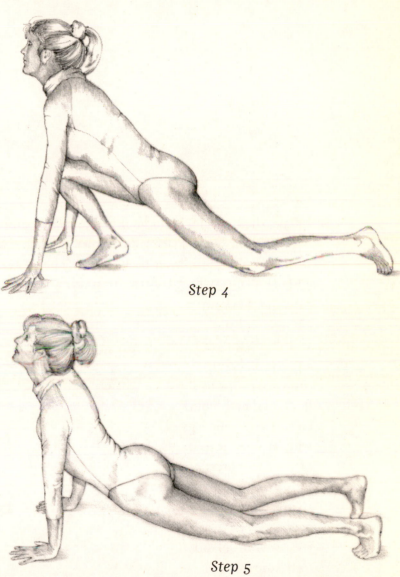

Step 4

Step 5

Vinyasa 1

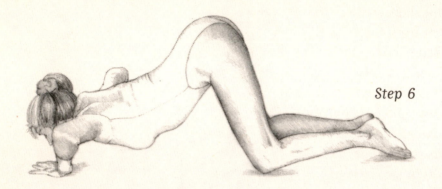

Step 6

6. Inhale, then exhale. Hold your breath as you drop to your knees and sit back on your heels. Place your elbows, chin, and chest on the floor; keep a strong arch in your lower back. (**Note:** This pose creates a lock over your adrenal glands, which control stress levels.)

7. Inhaling, lift your elbows, and slide your body forward and up. Exhaling, drop your hips to the floor, and arch your back. Keep your legs wide and the tops of your feet pressing into the floor. (**Note:** This pose creates a lock over your thymus gland to balance your immune system.)

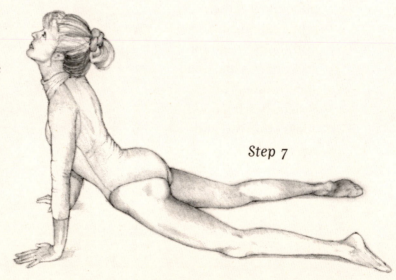

Step 7

8. Turn your toes under your feet for support. Exhaling, push up onto your feet and hands, drop your head between your shoulders, lift your hips toward the ceiling into an inverted "V" shape, and press your heels toward the floor. (**Note:** This pose puts pressure on your pineal and pituitary glands, which control appetite, sleep patterns, mood, sexuality, and intelligence. It also increases blood supply to your head for clear thinking and a clear complexion.)

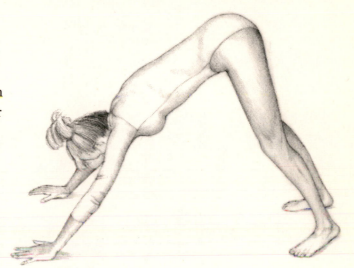

Step 8

9. Inhaling, step your left foot forward between your hands, bending your left leg into a lunge. Drop your right knee to the floor. Look forward, and lengthen through your chest.

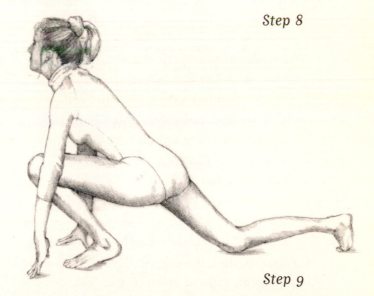

Step 9

Vinyasa 1

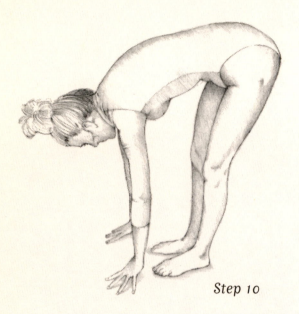

Step 10

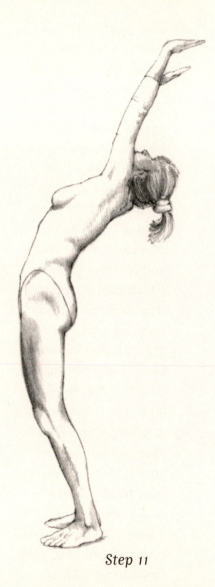

10. Exhaling, step your right foot forward to meet your left foot. Drop your upper body down toward your thighs, with your chin tucked under. Straighten both legs. (**Note:** This pose creates a lock in your thyroid gland, which controls your metabolic rate.)

11. Inhaling, stretch your arms forward; straighten up and raise your arms overhead; and arch backward strongly, with your head back. Exhaling, circle your arms wide, then bring them down to your sides.

Step 11

12. Inhaling, circle your arms wide out to the side, and join your palms overhead. Exhaling, bring your hands to your chest, palms together, fingers pointing up. Close your eyes. Inhale deeply and slowly, and release your hands to your sides.

13. Repeat the 12-step sequence 6 more times.

On completion of the Salute to the Sun,

➤ Stand quietly while your heart rate and breath return to normal.

➤ Lock your knees, and pull your abdominal muscles in.

➤ Tuck your buttocks under, and lift up through your rib cage while lengthening your spine.

➤ Lift your shoulders up, back, and down; your chin should be level with the floor.

➤ Lengthen your entire spine so that the vertebrae align themselves evenly. Imagine being pulled up by a string attached to the crown of your head.

➤ Hold this relaxed "perfect posture" pose for 7 Full Yoga Breaths (see Breathe on page 68 for detailed instructions), eyes closed, then open your eyes and relax.

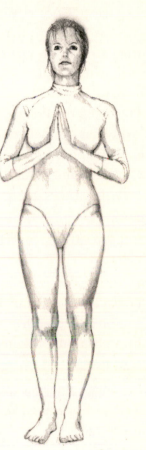

Step 12

Vinyasa 1

BREATHE

Present-Minded Awareness Breath

The regular practice of yoga teaches us that there is only the present moment, that time is a concept that exists solely in the imagination. The tendency to drift into past memories and future plans takes you away from yourself, making you insensitive to what is going on around you every moment of the day.

Practicing the Present-Minded Awareness Breath will help you learn to stay in the present, so that you can put all of your energy into working toward your goals. By keeping your energies on what you can do in the present, you get on with your life and reduce your worries about the future.

Benefits

Improves focus, concentration, and awareness of the need to stay in the moment

Focus

Practice moving your arms as slowly as you can, until you have the body and breath coordinated. Observe; stay in the moment of simply "being." Bring yourself back into each moment of each day, no matter how trivial your task.

1. Lie on the floor on your back with your arms at your sides, palms facing up, and legs extended, feet slightly apart. Inhaling, raise your arms above your head.
2. Exhaling, bring your arms down to the floor at your sides, while bending your right knee to your chest.
3. Inhaling, raise your arms overhead, palms facing up, while straightening your right leg parallel to the floor.
4. Repeat by slowly raising and lowering each alternate leg 6 times with the corresponding arm movements.

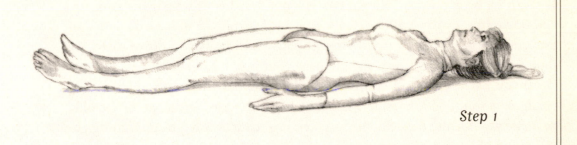

Step 1

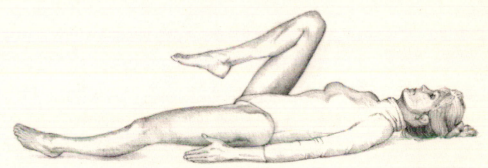

Step 2

6. Release and then draw your right knee to your chest. Loosely interlock your fingers around your knee.

7. Inhale slowly, and exhale 1½ times longer than your inhalation.

8. Repeat for a total of 7 slow breaths, then change legs. Repeat this breath with your left leg drawn into your chest.

9. Release your leg and lie quietly. Enjoy the feeling of being in the moment.

Present-Minded Awareness Breath

VISUALIZE

Creating a Healthy Self-Image

If you have been on the dieting merry-go-round and your weight has gone up and down like a yo-yo, you probably have felt frustrated and have despaired of ever reaching your ideal weight. These negative feelings have a life of their own; they tend to sap your energy and sabotage your best intentions.

If you have begun to read this book, then you have decided to make changes in your life. Choosing a healthier lifestyle means letting go of the old to make way for the new. So, the first step is to consciously practice letting go of the old ideas and habits that no longer work for you.

Benefits

Promotes the release of negative thoughts and their replacement with positive thoughts

Focus

Use your exhalation to release the tired, old self-limiting thoughts and your inhalation to energize the positive new thoughts and attitudes.

Relaxed Pose

1. Lie on the floor on your back with your arms by your sides, palms facing up, and feet flopped apart.
2. Inhale deeply through your nose; sigh as you exhale.
3. Inhaling deeply, expand and lift your abdomen, ribs, and chest.
4. Exhaling, consciously contract your abdomen first, then your ribs, and finally your chest, making sure you completely empty your lungs.
5. Take 6 more Full Yoga Breaths (see Breathe on page 68 for detailed instructions), and visualize the rise and fall of your chest with each breath.
6. Return to your own normal breathing pattern.

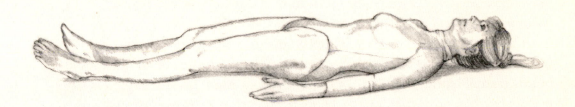

7. Inhaling deeply, think to yourself, "I am inhaling clarity."
8. Exhaling, think to yourself, "I am exhaling confusion."
9. Take 6 more Full Yoga Breaths. Each time, think the positive thought on the inhalation and the negative thought on the exhalation using the following ideas:

Positive Thought	Negative Thought
I am inhaling energy.	I am exhaling fatigue.
I am inhaling hope.	I am exhaling despair.
I am inhaling ease.	I am exhaling unease.
I am inhaling joy.	I am exhaling sadness.
I am inhaling lightness.	I am exhaling heaviness.
I am inhaling calmness.	I am exhaling anxiety.
I am inhaling self-assurance.	I am exhaling fear.

Creating a Healthy Self-Image

(**Note:** You can replace any of the suggested thoughts with your own. Energy always follows thought, and when you work positively with your breath to energize positive thoughts, the motivation and willpower will follow, enabling you to act on these positive thoughts.)

This breathing and visualization technique releases negative attitudes, thoughts and ideas so that you can create some space in your mind. As a result of this mental "spring cleaning," you may become aware that something is lacking in your life, no matter how much material, family, or career "wealth" you enjoy. Anxiety, fatigue, or stress may mask this sense of lack. It may come out as dissatisfaction and despair with your life. Are you using food as a channel to release the pent-up frustration of unfulfilled ambitions, desires, and aspirations? Are you eating out of boredom? Unhealthy eating habits often are a result of unfulfilled creative energy wrongly channeled into a desire for food. As you practice this technique, observe what comes into your consciousness, and be aware of any sense of lacking or emptiness.

After you have completed the visualization exercise, reflect on the following questions:

➤ What parts of my life are missing?
➤ Which roles could be more developed?

If you keep getting messages that remind you of unfulfilled desires, ambitions, or aspirations, don't ignore them. Recurring messages can guide you in making your life more fulfilling. Keep expanding your roles and skills so you can adapt and design your life to give it more balance and harmony. Keep asking yourself, "How whole is my life?" and find a structure that supports your self-growth and self-development. In this way, as your life becomes more satisfying, your dependence on food as a source of satisfaction will diminish.

chapter five

Routine 2

Routine 2 is more challenging than Routine 1. It builds strength in all the muscles and joints of the body with deep lunges and a variation of the Salute to the Sun. The poses convey several benefits:

➤ **Lunge in Prayer** stretches and opens up your hips so that exercising becomes easier and more enjoyable. The more easily your body moves, the more you will want to keep moving, which will speed up your metabolic rate throughout the day.

➤ **Mountain Pose** increases your awareness of how to correct poor posture, which can make you look heavier and older.

➤ **Cleansing Breath** is recommended by the Bihar School of Yoga in India to reduce gas and constipation while toning the digestive organs.

➤ **Vinyasa 2** requires you to jump your feet back and support your body strongly on your arms, which improves bone and muscle strength. The strong arch in your lower back strengthens your back muscles to improve your posture.

➤ **Full Yoga Breath** forms the basis for many yoga poses and ensures that you get the maximum amount of oxygen into every cell of your body to nourish and repair cell tissues.

➤ **Affirm Your Existing Qualities** is a visualization to help reprogram your mind with positive thoughts about who you are.

Did You Know?

It takes about 3,500 calories to make 1 pound of fat. The average person would need to walk for about 11.5 hours to burn off 3,500 calories—or 1 pound of fat. If you combine 30 minutes of a dynamic vinyasa with a brisk 30-minute walk (3.5–4 miles an hour) each day, you will complete 28 hours of aerobic-type exercise a month. This regime could lead to a safe weight loss of more than 2 pounds of fat a month. If you also eat fewer calories, the loss will be even greater.

STRETCH AND TONE

Lunge in Prayer

Benefits

Stretches and tones the upper thighs and pelvic floor muscles; opens up the hips

Focus

Keep your back straight and upright, and relax your shoulders.

1. Kneel on the floor. Step your right foot forward into a lunge.
2. Place both hands on your right thigh, one hand over the other.
3. Move your weight forward and backward a couple of times until you are in a fully extended lunge; adjust the placement of your right foot if necessary.
4. Bring your hands together in front of your chest, palms together, fingers pointing up.
5. Inhale a Full Yoga Breath (see BREATHE section in this chapter). Exhaling, consciously let all of your body weight come down evenly through your groin, stretching your inner thighs. Continue inhaling and exhaling for 4 breaths, sinking a little lower into the lunge with each exhalation.
6. Bring your right foot back to the kneeling position.
7. Step your left foot forward into a lunge. Repeat the pose on your left side, first with hands on your thigh, then with palms together in front of your chest, fingers pointing up. Hold for 4 complete breaths.
8. Bring your left foot back to the kneeling position, and relax.

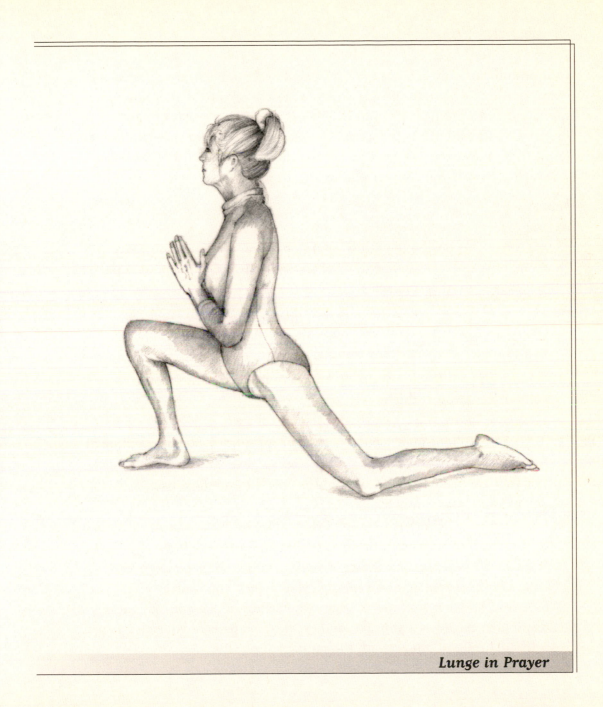

Lunge in Prayer

IMPROVE POSTURE

Mountain Pose

Poor posture not only contributes to back and neck problems over the years; it also can add 10 years to the way you look. Rounded shoulders, a hunched spine, and a protruding belly immediately age a person, whereas upright shoulders, a straight spine, and a firm abdomen typify vitality and youthfulness. Improve your awareness of good posture by checking and adjusting your posture each time you find yourself waiting in a line.

Benefits

Improves posture; improves sense of balance

(**Note:** This pose, often called "perfect posture," will make you very aware of your body alignment. To check your posture in the pose, stand sideways in front of a mirror.)

Focus

Center your weight evenly over both feet. Keep your tailbone slightly tucked under and your spine elongated.

1. Stand with your feet hip-width apart and your arms resting at your sides, palms on your outer thighs.
2. Lock your knees, and contract your abdominal muscles.
3. Tuck your tailbone under, and stretch your spine from its base up through the top of your head.
4. Lift your rib cage up; lift your shoulders up, then roll them backward and down, away from your neck.
5. Lengthen your neck as if you were being pulled up by a piece of string tied to the crown of your head. Bring your chin level with the floor.
6. Relax in the pose. Become aware of where your weight is placed over your feet. (Is it coming down through your arches, your outer feet, your heels, or your toes?) Adjust your stance so that your weight is distributed evenly over your feet and evenly to all parts of your feet, so your soles are firmly in contact with the earth.

7. Close your eyes, and stand perfectly still. Hold the pose for 7 Full Yoga Breaths (see BREATHE section in this chapter).

8. Open your eyes. Check your posture in the mirror.

9. Repeat the pose while balancing a book on your head. Hold the pose for 7 breaths.

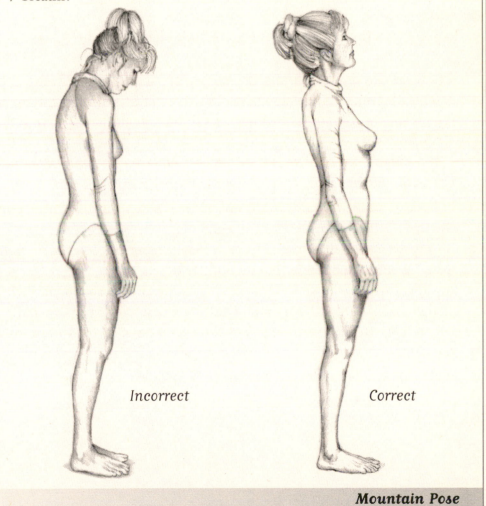

Incorrect　　　　　*Correct*

Mountain Pose

IMPROVE DIGESTION AND ELIMINATION

Cleansing Breath

When the body is constipated, it retains water to dilute the toxins. Bloating occurs, which results in increased weight. The Bihar School of Yoga in India recommends practicing the Cleansing Breath to reduce bloating and constipation.

Benefits
Reduced constipation and bloating; tones the digestive organs

Focus
Your breathing should resemble the panting of a dog. Visualize your abdomen becoming firmer and flatter as a result of increasing the strength of your abdominal muscles that move food throughout the digestive and eliminatory systems.

Warnings: Practice on an empty stomach. This exercise is not recommended for people with high blood pressure, heart problems, or peptic ulcers.

1. Sit back on your heels with your hands resting loosely on your knees; lean slightly forward. Keep your arms straight.
2. Open your mouth slightly, and let your tongue hang out. Keep your mouth open (i.e., breathe through your mouth) for this exercise.
3. Inhaling, expand your abdomen; exhaling, contract your abdomen. Quickly alternate inhalation and exhalation (with accompanying expansion and contraction), strongly activating your abdominal muscles, for 10 breaths.
4. Rest.
5. Repeat the Cleansing Breath for another 10 breaths.

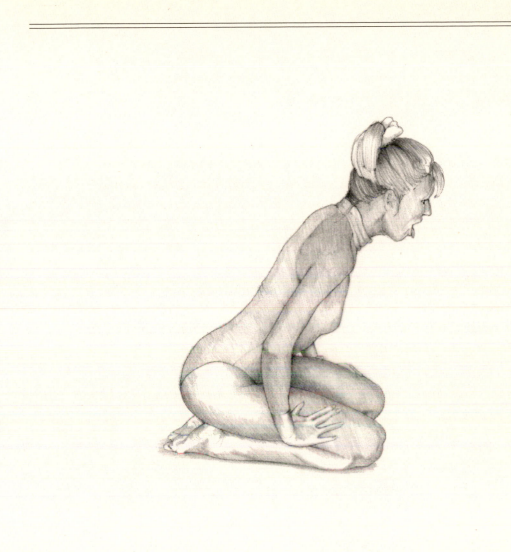

Cleansing Breath

IMPROVE METABOLIC RATE

Vinyasa 2

This variation of Salute to the Sun is a more challenging sequence than Vinyasa 1 because you jump your feet back instead of stepping them back. The 13 steps can be practiced as fast or as slowly as you like.

Benefits

Stretches and tones all muscles and joints, strengthens bones, improves breathing rate and heart rate, increases energy level, improves concentration, cleanses the glandular system of toxins, lifts depression and anxiety, speeds metabolic rate for weight maintenance

Focus

Keep your movements smooth and graceful; maintain even and rhythmic breathing.

Warning: If you experience chronic back pain or have injured your back, consult a yoga instructor before proceeding with this vinyasa.

I. Stand with your feet hip-width apart and your hands in front of your chest, palms together, fingers pointing up. Inhaling, lift your arms to the side, to shoulder height.

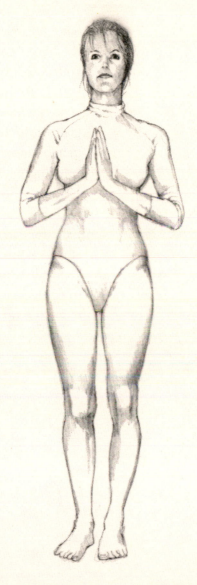

Step 1

Vinyasa 2

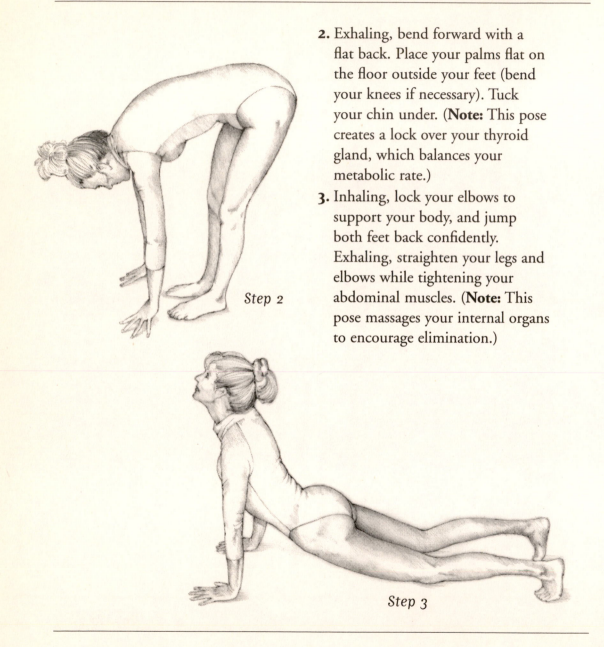

2. Exhaling, bend forward with a flat back. Place your palms flat on the floor outside your feet (bend your knees if necessary). Tuck your chin under. (**Note:** This pose creates a lock over your thyroid gland, which balances your metabolic rate.)

3. Inhaling, lock your elbows to support your body, and jump both feet back confidently. Exhaling, straighten your legs and elbows while tightening your abdominal muscles. (**Note:** This pose massages your internal organs to encourage elimination.)

Step 2

Step 3

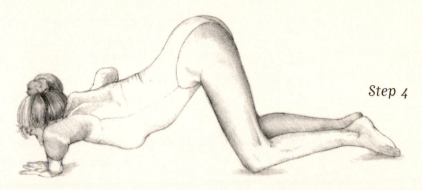

Step 4

4. Inhale, then exhale. Hold your breath as you drop to your knees and sit back on your heels. Place your chin and chest on the floor and lift your elbows; keep a strong arch in your lower back. (**Note:** This pose creates a lock over your adrenal glands, which control stress levels.)

5. Inhaling, slide your body forward and up. Exhaling, drop your hips to the floor, and arch your back. Keep your legs wide and the tops of your feet pressing into the floor. (**Note:** This pose creates a lock over your thymus gland to balance your immune system.)

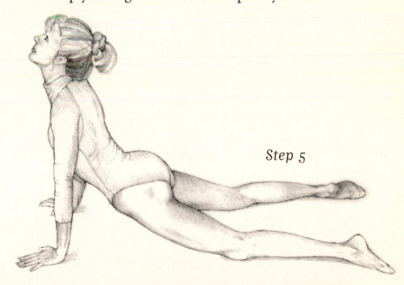

Step 5

Vinyasa 2

6. Inhaling, tuck your toes under and bring your feet close together. Exhaling, straighten your arms to lift your upper body and hips off the floor. Keep your legs straight. Arch your back strongly, and stretch up through your chest. Imagine that you are trying to push your hips through your elbows to increase the arch in your back. Hold this pose for 2 breaths.

(**Note:** This pose creates a lock over your thymus gland to improve immune system function.)

Step 6

7. Inhale. Exhaling, push up onto your feet and hands, drop your head between your shoulders, lift your hips to the ceiling to create an inverted "V" shape, and press your heels toward the floor to stretch your hamstrings.

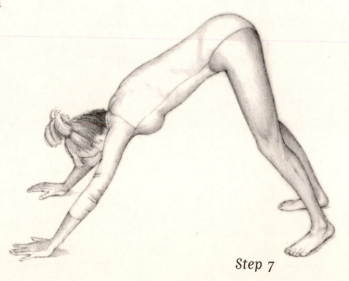

Step 7

8. Inhaling, step your left foot forward between your hands, bending your left leg into a lunge. Drop your right knee to the floor. Look forward, and lengthen through your chest.

9. Exhaling and maintaining your leg position, straighten your back. Place your hands on your thighs. Rest both hands on your left thigh, one on top of the other.

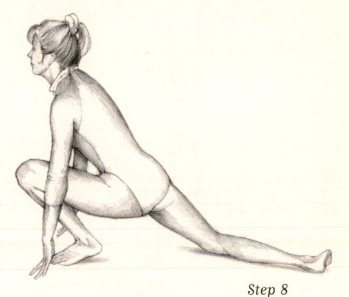

Step 8

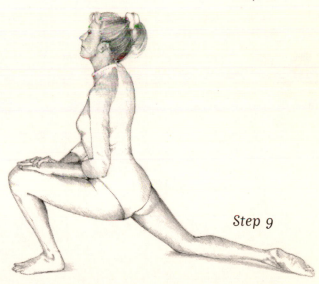

Step 9

Vinyasa 2

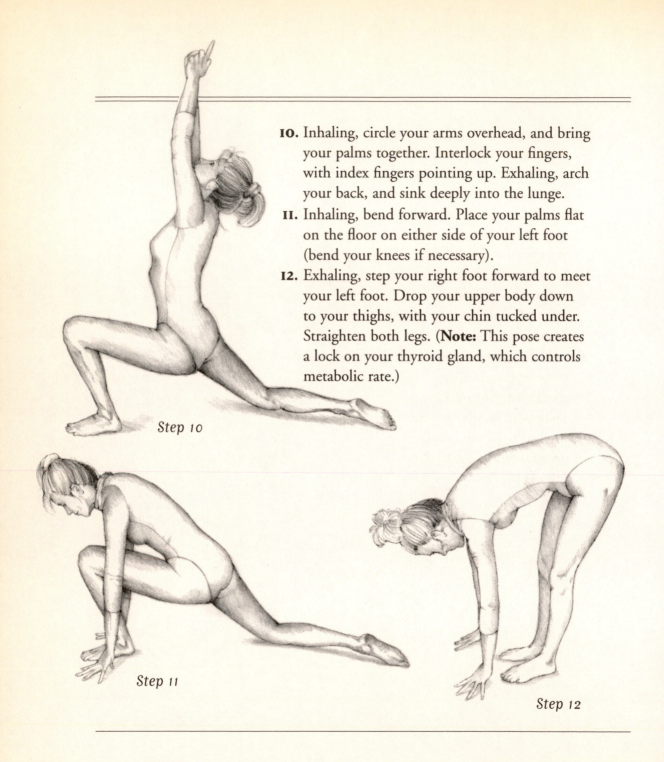

10. Inhaling, circle your arms overhead, and bring your palms together. Interlock your fingers, with index fingers pointing up. Exhaling, arch your back, and sink deeply into the lunge.

11. Inhaling, bend forward. Place your palms flat on the floor on either side of your left foot (bend your knees if necessary).

12. Exhaling, step your right foot forward to meet your left foot. Drop your upper body down to your thighs, with your chin tucked under. Straighten both legs. (**Note:** This pose creates a lock on your thyroid gland, which controls metabolic rate.)

Step 10

Step 11

Step 12

13. Inhaling, come up with a straight back, and lift your arms to the side to shoulder height. Exhaling, bring your hands together in front of your chest, palms together, fingers pointing up. Close your eyes. Inhale deeply and slowly, and release your hands to your sides.

14. Complete the sequence 6 times, alternating sides with each leg in the lunge.

15. Return to Mountain Pose. Hold for 7 Full Yoga Breaths (see BREATHE section in this chapter).

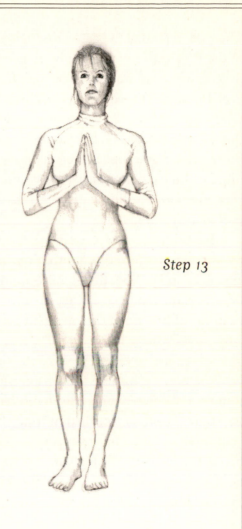

Step 13

Vinyasa 2

BREATHE

Full Yoga Breath

The Full Yoga Breath is used throughout many of yoga poses because it uses all of the lung capacity for maximum energy. Deep breathing techniques increase oxygen supply to nourish every cell in the body. The body's response to an overabundance of oxygen in the blood is to slow down respiration rate and brain function, to allow carbon dioxide levels to return to normal. During this time, the mind and body become very quiet. You can experience this stillness for moments at a time during your yoga routines. With simple breathing techniques, you can take yourself down into that deep velvety darkness behind the eyes and, in the stillness, practice listening to what is to be revealed to you moment by moment.

Breathing techniques train your mind to tune out outside stimuli and to focus your energy and concentration, which has a calming effect. The less anxious you become, the more you can detach yourself from all those busy-yet-unimportant thoughts and regain a sense of control. The more you practice deep breathing, the more energized your thoughts will become, and the more empowered you will feel.

Babies automatically practice the Full Yoga Breath, because this is the way we were born to breathe. Unfortunately, because of poor posture and rushing to meet deadlines, adults have forgotten how to breathe naturally and effortlessly. Many people sit slouched in front of the television, hunched in front of the computer, or clutching a steering wheel for much of the day. These poor sitting habits compress the diaphragm and lead to shallow breathing, with resultant neck and shoulder pain. Most adults take breathing for granted and do not breathe consciously or use their entire lung capacity.

Benefits

Improves concentration, energy levels, resistance to disease and infection, circulation, capacity to manage stress, and ability to switch off mentally; if practiced regularly with relaxation and visualization techniques, eliminates cravings and dependency on health-destroying substances such as nicotine, alcohol, sugar, and excess fats

Focus

Consciously release and expand your diaphragm to allow more oxygen into your lungs.

Warnings: Although you may become a little dizzy the first few times you practice this technique, the feeling will pass with time and practice. Breathing techniques can be quite taxing on your lungs if you are normally a shallow breather, so start gradually. Even a few minutes a day is beneficial. With practice, the time can be increased safely if you follow a few common-sense guidelines:

➤ *If you suffer from hypertension, do not strain by making your inhalations and exhalations too deep. If you feel any discomfort, stop and rest for a while before continuing.*

➤ *If your head becomes hot, lie down in a relaxed position to rest for a few minutes to recover from the strain.*

➤ *More is not necessarily better. If you feel dizzy or lightheaded, stop immediately and return to your normal breathing pattern.*

Full Yoga Breath

STAGE 1

Focus

On the inhalation, allow the area around your navel to balloon up; on the exhalation, expel all of your breath to prepare your lungs for the next inhalation.

1. Lie on the floor on your back with your arms at your sides, palms facing up, and feet flopped apart. Begin to pay attention to your breath.

2. Ask yourself the following questions:

   ➤ Does my breath feel stuck around the middle of my abdomen or in the top of my chest? (Release any tightness with the exhalation.)

   ➤ Are my inhalations the same length as my exhalations? (Make them both even.)

   ➤ Am I straining on the inhalation or the exhalation? (Don't force the breath; relax into the breathing.)

3. Slowly inhaling through your nose for a count of 4, expand your lower abdomen up, as though you were releasing a tight belt across your tummy. Feel the lower part of your lungs expand and fill with air.

4. Exhaling for a count of 4, consciously pull your abdominal muscles back down slowly to flatten your abdomen.

5. Repeat the inhalation and exhalation 3 times.

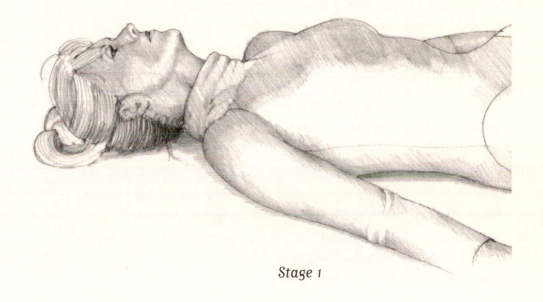

Stage 1

Full Yoga Breath

STAGE 2

Focus

Stretch the tiny muscles between each rib bone, so your ribs can lift up and sideways.

6. Inhaling slowly for a count of 4, expand your lower abdomen.
7. Continue breathing for 2 more counts, and widen your ribs up and sideways. Feel the middle part of your lungs fill with air.
8. Exhaling for a count of 6, flatten your abdomen, then your ribs.
9. Repeat the inhalation and exhalation 3 times.

STAGE 3

Focus

Make the movement of your abdomen, ribs, and upper chest smooth and rhythmic, without strain—like the ebb and flow of waves on a beach. Relax as you exhale as slowly as possible.

10. Inhaling slowly, expand your abdomen and ribs for a total count of 6.
11. Inhaling for another count, expand your upper chest muscles just under your collarbone. Feel the top part of your lungs fill with air.
12. Exhaling for a count of 7, feel first your abdomen, then your ribs, and finally the top of your chest empty of air.
13. Repeat the inhalation and exhalation 3 times.

COMPLETE

14. Combining Stages 1–3, practice 7 rounds of Full Yoga Breath, inhaling and exhaling for a count of 7 each time.
15. Return to your normal breathing pattern.

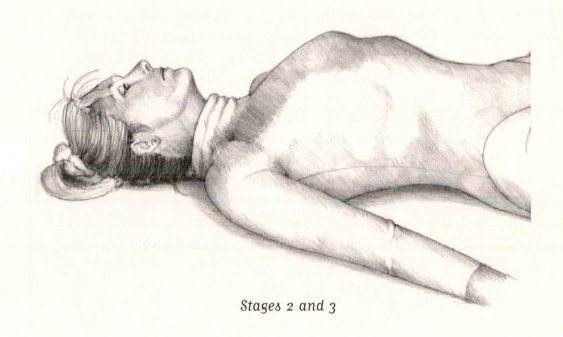

Stages 2 and 3

Because the Full Yoga Breath is so integral to yoga practice, a few points are worth noting:

- This is not a race, so do not rush your progress. Take time to become familiar with your breathing pattern; it is unique to you. With practice, it will become one of your most important tools for maximizing health and well-being.

- Full Yoga Breath is best practiced lying down initially, until it becomes rhythmic and easy. When the technique becomes easier, it can be practiced standing or seated.

- The best time to practice this breath is on waking, when your body is relaxed. If you struggle to get out of bed each morning, try this breath 7 times on waking. As your body fills with oxygen and your brain becomes energized, you should find it much easier to become active.

- At first, this technique may feel awkward. It takes time to undo bad breathing habits. Initially, exaggerate the movement of your chest, to experience the full expansion and contraction of your lungs as they fill with air. The breath will become quieter with practice.

- This deep breathing technique is used when practicing many yoga poses: gather the energy within on the inhalation, and extend and stretch into a pose on the exhalation.

- Do not be alarmed if you feel a little dizzy after completing this breathing technique. Make the counts a little faster until you feel more comfortable. It may take time for your brain to get used to the increased oxygen supply if your breathing is normally shallow.

Full Yoga Breath

VISUALIZE

Affirm Existing Qualities

You have everything in your physical body and personality to do all the things that you came to do in this life. Sometimes we lose track of the very best in ourselves throughout the busy-ness of the day, which makes us doubt our abilities and causes unfounded anxiety. This visualization exercise will put you firmly back in touch with the very best of yourself, to reassure you that you have all the tools you need to achieve all your goals in life.

All living things contain a life force, or prana. Practicing breathing with awareness increases the flow of prana to all the cells in the body. In this exercise, first use the Etheric Breath to energize each of your most powerful personality traits. Then, visualize the personality traits that you would like to have and to affirm that you are becoming the person you would like to be.

Benefits
Energizes the body; creates a sense of self-sufficiency

Focus
Consciously use your breath to affirm and energize your most positive personality traits.

STAGE 1

Cross-Legged Position

1. Sit on the floor in Cross-Legged Position. (**Note:** If this position is not comfortable, sit on a folded towel to tilt your hips forward and take the pressure off your knees. Alternatively, sit with your legs stretched out in front, leaning against a wall if necessary, or sit in a chair.) Have a pen and a piece of paper within arm's reach.

2. Take 7 Full Yoga Breaths (see BREATHE section in this chapter). In a very detached way, watch your breath settle.

3. Reflect for a moment on what you believe to be your seven strongest and best personality traits (e.g., generosity, ability to give and receive love, sensitivity, empathy, and so on). Write them down.

4. Following your breath, relax your shoulders. Become conscious of the rhythm of your breath.

5. Expand your diaphragm on the inhalation and contract it on the exhalation, as if you are loosening and tightening a belt around your abdominal area.

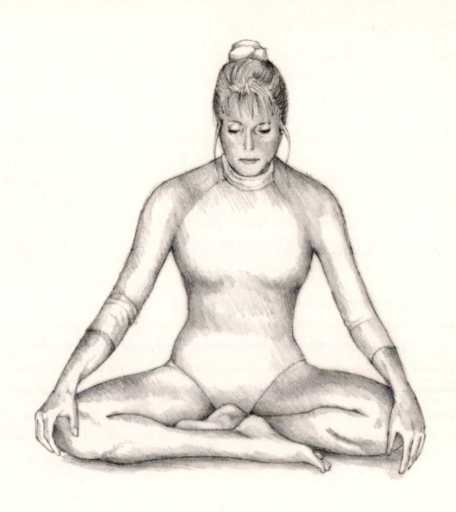

Etheric Breath

6. Begin the Etheric Breath. Inhaling, imagine that you are drawing in a stream of golden energy through the crown of your head.

7. Hold your breath; mentally take this energy to your heart, solar plexus, spleen, and back to your heart in a triangle 3 times. Imagine that you are charging your breath with the energy from each of these powerful centers in your body.

8. Exhaling, affirm to yourself your first trait. For example, if the first trait on your list is "generosity," then think to yourself "I am generous" as you exhale. Feel the power behind your breath energizing this thought.

9. Inhaling, imagine drawing golden energy down through the crown of your head.

10. Hold your breath; mentally take this energy to your heart, solar plexus, spleen, and back to your heart in a triangle 3 times.

11. Exhaling, affirm to yourself the second personality trait on your list.

12. Repeat this sequence with each of the remaining personality traits.

13. Sit quietly and breathe normally, mentally acknowledging all of the wonderful personality traits within you.

(**Note:** Take the time to feel the energy behind each of these affirmations confirming who and what you are. Feel very powerful and inwardly self-assured with each energizing thought as you exhale.)

STAGE 2

Know that you must first see in order to become. Before you can make any positive changes in your life, you must be able to clearly visualize those changes. This ability to see yourself as you would like to be requires practice and perseverance. In the beginning, it does not matter if you only think the thoughts rather than see the visual images.

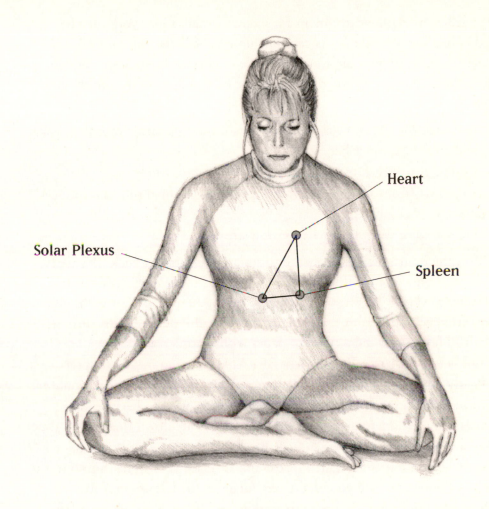

Heart

Solar Plexus

Spleen

To create the right environment for mental visualization, you must be relaxed enough so your thoughts can flow unimpeded without your critical, judgmental self getting in the way. This state of detached relaxation can be greatly enhanced by using one or more of the following tools during the next exercise:

> rhythmic breathing, to change your brain wave patterns from the logical alpha to the creative beta;
> soothing, unstructured music to help your mind drift;
> an aroma (from a scented candle, incense, or essential oil) that induces pleasant memories; or
> the sound of water (rain, waves, or a stream).

1. Sit on the floor in Cross-Legged Position, with a straight back. (**Note:** If this position is not comfortable, sit on a folded towel to tilt your hips forward and take the pressure off your knees. Alternatively, sit with your legs stretched out in front, leaning against a wall if necessary, or sit in a chair.) Have a pen and a piece of paper within arm's reach.

2. Complete 7 Full Yoga Breaths (see BREATHE section in this chapter).

3. Quietly reflect for a moment on seven personality traits that you would like to strengthen in your life. For example, you may wish to become more patient, more understanding, or more loving. Write down these seven traits.

4. Begin 7 rounds of Alternate Nostril Breathing (see Routine 7 in Chapter 10 for an illustration and detailed instructions). Place your right thumb to the right of your nose and your right ring finger to the left of your nose.

5. Close your right nostril with your thumb, and inhale through your left nostril.

6. Close your left nostril with your ring finger, open your right nostril, and exhale through your right nostril.

7. Inhale through your right nostril, close your right nostril, open your left nostril, and exhale through your left nostril. (This is the completion of one round of Alternate Nostril Breathing. In each round, you exhale twice—once through each nostril.) Practice 7 more rounds of Alternate Nostril Breathing to complete one set of Alternate Nostril Breathing.

8. Next, complete a set of 7 rounds of Alternate Nostril Breathing with affirmations. During the first round, affirm to yourself your first desired trait on each of the two exhalations. For instance, if you would like to become more loving, think to yourself, "I am becoming more and more and more loving" as you exhale. Continue Alternate Nostril Breathing until you have affirmed each of the seven personality traits, twice per round.

9. Release your hand back to your lap, and sit quietly, visualizing yourself as possessing the desired personality traits. See the way you would speak, act, and think with these desired traits.

(**Note:** You do not have to believe these affirmations to begin with; practice repeating the affirmations. Eventually, they will become deeply ingrained in your subconscious mind. You then will begin to act as if you already have these desired qualities. This is the magic of affirmations!)

chapter six

Routine 3

Routine 3 firms up and tones your abdominal muscles, improves your eliminatory system to prevent constipation and bloating, and thus will help to prevent increased fat storage on your abdomen. The poses convey several benefits:

➤ **Buttocks Walking** activates all of your abdominal muscles to improve muscle tone, firm your abdomen, and make your buttocks more shapely.

➤ **Star Stretch** firms and tones your abdominal muscles and improves circulation to the abdominal area.

➤ **Raised Stomach Lift** increases circulation to your liver, kidneys, and stomach to improve their function. It also opens up the emotional center around your solar plexus, promoting a feeling of trust and openness, which transmutes to everyone you come in contact with. This relaxed acceptance of yourself leaves you feeling nurtured from within and releases your need to use food as a source of comfort or nurturing.

➤ **Vinyasa 3** improves the strength and flexibility of the muscles and joints in your arms and legs as you make repeated jumps into the air. The vibration on your bones as your legs hit the floor (i.e., weight-bearing exercise) encourages your bones to retain calcium and stay strong. Jumping in the air also

Did You Know?

An excess of abdominal fat is detrimental to your health because of the increased risk of heart disease. However, extra fat on your hips and thighs may actually protect your heart.

gets you in touch with that playful childlike aspect of yourself, reminding you not to take life too seriously. This vinyasa also boosts your metabolic rate.

➤ **Anti-Anxiety Breath** helps to avoid overbreathing throughout the day. Overbreathing causes you to sigh and strain with your breath, making you feel anxious. As you learn to completely empty your lungs, you will feel emptiness in your emotions and your mind. It teaches you the sheer pleasure of taking a deep, full breath when your lungs are completely empty. This breath often leads you to a quiet place where you will have few or no thoughts momentarily; it often is used as a prelude to entering a meditative state.

➤ **A Visit to a Wise Old Woman** is a visualization that quiets your mind so that you can tune into all of your intuitive wisdom about how to heal your body. This wisdom is always available, but it often gets lost in the busy-ness of your day, or you choose to ignore the messages— to your own detriment.

STRETCH AND TONE

Buttocks Walking

Benefits

Strengthens the abdominal muscles

Focus

Create a fast-paced rhythm, and get as much lift and movement as possible for maximum benefit. Visualize your body building up lots of heat as you breathe deeply to increase your metabolic rate and temperature.

(**Note:** Buttocks Walking is best practiced on a smooth, hard floor.)

1. Sit on the floor with your legs stretched out in front of you, and clasp your elbows with your hands.
2. Lift your right buttock off the floor by bending your right knee, and slide your right heel forward a few inches.
3. Lift your left buttock off the floor by bending your left knee, and slide your left heel forward a few inches.
4. Alternate lifting and lowering your buttocks to "walk" yourself to the other side of the room.
5. When you can go no farther, put it in reverse: "walk" backward on your buttocks to your starting point.
6. Repeat another forward-and-backward "walk" across the room. Swing your clasped elbows vigorously from side to side to help build up momentum. Build up speed as you move along, and keep breathing vigorously.
7. Stop, sit, and relax.

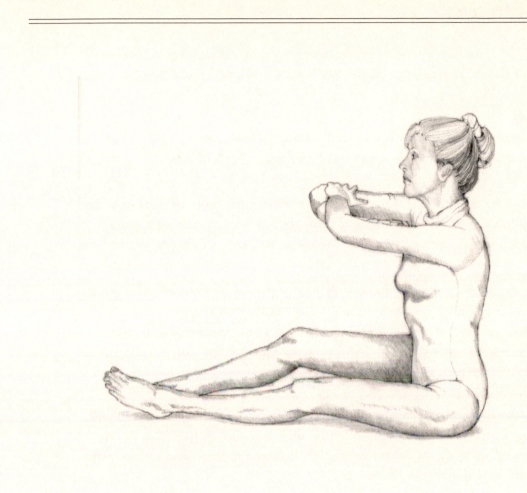

Buttocks Walking

IMPROVE POSTURE

Star Stretch

The act of consciously tensing and releasing your muscles makes you more aware of the difference between the two and of how good relaxation can feel.

Benefits
Improves circulation to the abdominal area; releases tension across the abdomen, chest, and back to make breathing easier and deeper

Focus
Focus on extending and tensing every muscle, even those of your face. As you tense your muscles, visualize your body as being as taut as a guitar string. As you release the tension, visualize yourself as being as soft as a rag doll.

1. Lie on the floor on your back with your arms and legs spread wide, palms facing up; your body should resemble the shape of a starfish.
2. Inhale deeply, then exhale. Hold your breath for 7 counts as you stretch and lengthen through your arms, pressing the backs of your hands into the floor. Leave your legs soft.
3. Release and relax.
4. Inhale, then exhale. Hold your breath for a count of 7 as you stretch and lengthen through your legs while pointing your toes to the floor. Leave your upper body soft. Press your lower back to the floor, and tighten your abdominal muscles and buttocks.
5. Release and relax.
6. Inhale, then exhale. Hold your breath for 7 counts as you stretch through your right arm and left leg diagonally through your body, pointing your toes and fingers.

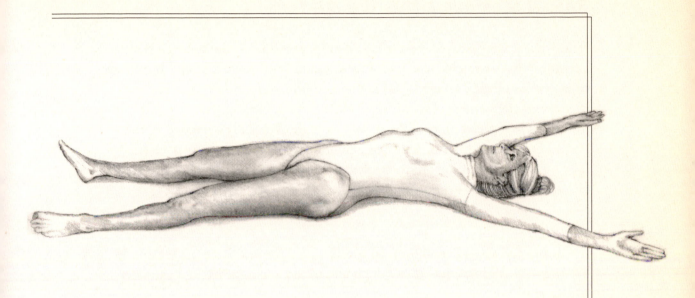

7. Release and relax.

8. Inhale, then exhale. Hold your breath for 7 counts as you stretch through your left arm and right leg diagonally through your body, pointing your toes and fingers. Exhale and relax.

9. Inhale, then exhale. Hold your breath for 7 counts, as you stretch through your arms and legs. Flatten the backs of your hands and your back to the floor, and tighten every muscle in your body, including those of your face.

10. Relax by practicing 3 Full Yoga Breaths (see Breathe on page 68 for detailed instructions).

Star Stretch

IMPROVE DIGESTION AND ELIMINATION

Raised Stomach Lift with Bent Legs

When negative thoughts and feelings dominate our lives, the solar plexus can become very tense. This tension limits our emotional responses and breathing capacity. Resulting shallow breathing and emotional tension can upset our digestive system and lead to constipation.

As tense muscles around the solar plexus are physically stretched in the Raised Stomach Lift with Bent Legs, emotional blockages can be released. The breath then can flow more freely, and the function of the digestive and eliminatory systems is improved.

Benefits

Tones and firms the abdominal muscles and buttocks; releases tension in the solar plexus; strengthens the bones of the wrists, arms, and shoulders

Focus

Concentrate on the feelings of release, openness, and trust, which you can bring into your personal relationships to make them more meaningful.

1. Lie on the floor on your back with your feet flat on the floor on either side of your hips, as close to your buttocks as possible. Clasp your ankles firmly, pulling them close to your buttocks, then lift your ankles and come up onto your toes.

2. Squeeze your shoulder blades together, and lift your hips to the ceiling. Arch your back strongly, and move your weight onto your shoulder blades.

3. Place the crown of your head on the floor.

4. Cup your palms behind your waist, fingertips pointing toward your spine. Wriggle from shoulder to shoulder, and move your elbows closer together under your back to form a stronger arch.

5. Flatten the back of your neck, and distribute your weight evenly between your neck and shoulders.

6. Hold the pose steady, then flatten your feet.

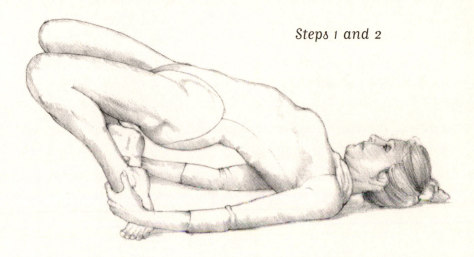

Steps 1 and 2

7. Inhale through your nose, then exhale forcefully through your mouth. Holding your breath, pull your abdominal muscles in firmly, and squeeze your buttocks together. Hold the tension for a count of 7.

8. Inhale deeply and slowly, then exhale.

9. Inhale through your nose, and exhale forcefully through your mouth. Holding your breath, pull your abdominal muscles in firmly, and squeeze your buttocks together. Hold the tension for a count of 14.

10. Breathe slowly, in and out. Repeat the sequence again, but this time hold the tension for a count of 21.

11. Slide your elbows out, and lower your hips to the floor. Straighten your legs, and rest with your arms at your sides, palms facing up, feet flopped apart. Breathe deeply, feeling a sense of release and inner strength throughout your abdomen.

Raised Stomach Lift with Bent Legs

IMPROVE METABOLIC RATE

Vinyasa 3

By bringing your head lower than your heart in part of this sequence, your heart gets a rest and your head receives extra blood circulation.

Benefits

Improves strength and flexibility of the arms and legs; clears complexion; improves memory and focus

Focus

Keep your movements smooth and graceful; maintain deep, even, and rhythmic breathing.

1. Stand with your feet hip-width apart. Bring your hands to the front of your chest, fingertips together and palms facing down.

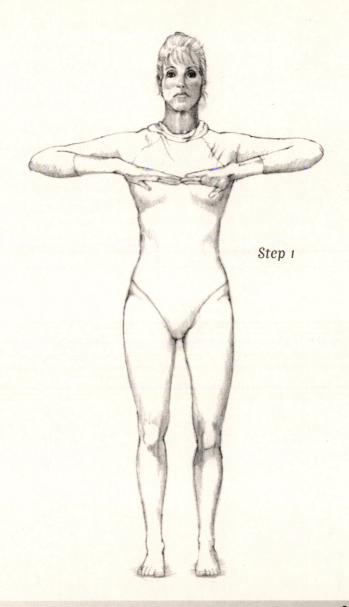

Step 1

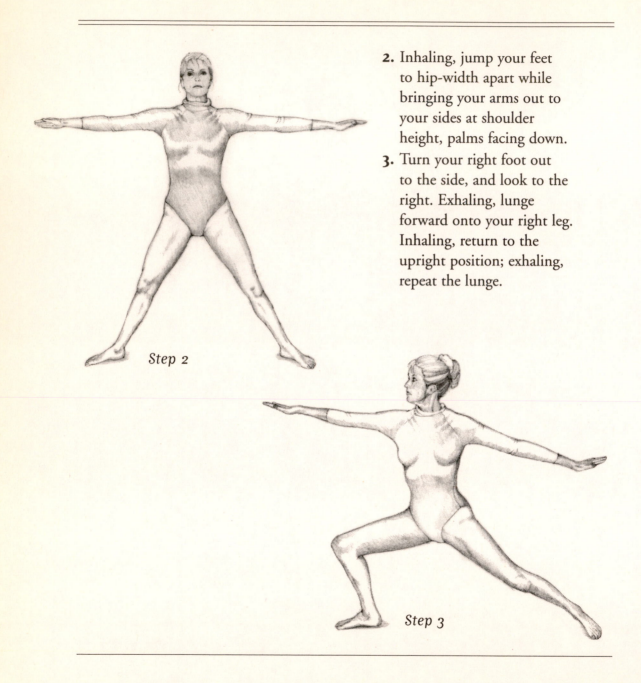

2. Inhaling, jump your feet to hip-width apart while bringing your arms out to your sides at shoulder height, palms facing down.

3. Turn your right foot out to the side, and look to the right. Exhaling, lunge forward onto your right leg. Inhaling, return to the upright position; exhaling, repeat the lunge.

Step 2

Step 3

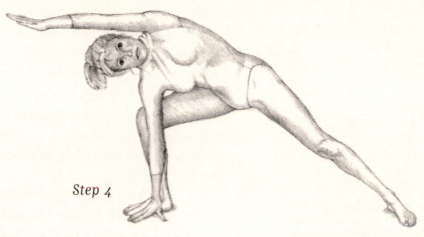

Step 4

4. Inhaling, return to the upright position; exhaling, lunge a third time. Place your right palm flat on the floor, inside your right foot. Bring your left arm straight over your head, close to your ear. Pull your left shoulder back to a point of resistance.

5. Inhaling, return to an upright position while lifting your arms to shoulder height, palms facing down. Turn the right foot back in.

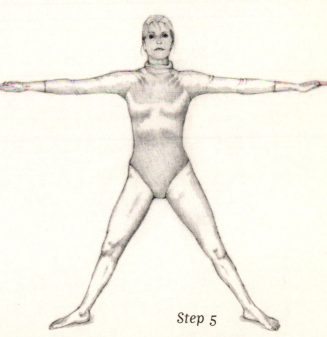

Step 5

Vinyasa 3

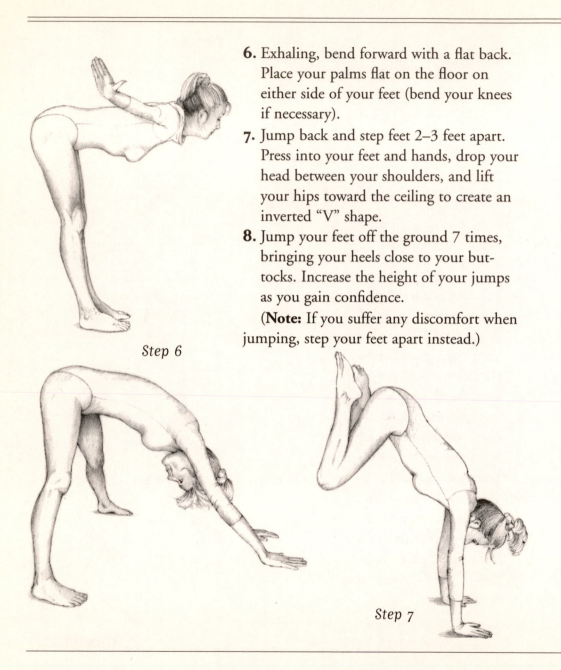

6. Exhaling, bend forward with a flat back. Place your palms flat on the floor on either side of your feet (bend your knees if necessary).

7. Jump back and step feet 2–3 feet apart. Press into your feet and hands, drop your head between your shoulders, and lift your hips toward the ceiling to create an inverted "V" shape.

8. Jump your feet off the ground 7 times, bringing your heels close to your buttocks. Increase the height of your jumps as you gain confidence.

(**Note:** If you suffer any discomfort when jumping, step your feet apart instead.)

Step 6

Step 7

9. On the last jump, land with your feet 4–6 feet apart on the floor. "Walk" your hands back until they are under your shoulders, then make two fists on the floor. Step your feet in, close to your hands.

10. Inhaling, stand up while lifting your arms out to your sides at shoulder height; exhaling, bring your hands to your chest, fingertips together and palms facing down.

11. Inhale deeply and slowly, then repeat the sequence 6 more times. Alternate lunging to the side in each sequence.

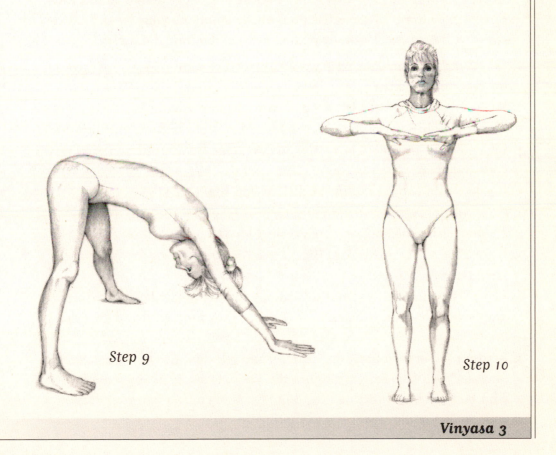

Step 9

Step 10

Vinyasa 3

BREATHE

Anti-Anxiety Breath

By practicing the Anti-Anxiety Breath, you consciously empty your lungs of stale air and your bloodstream of excess carbon dioxide, which can leave you feeling irritable, fatigued, and anxious. You then can inhale deeply, naturally replenishing your energy and restoring your well-being with fresh air.

Benefits

Relieves anxiety, fatigue, and irritability

Focus

Do not rush; resist the temptation to inhale for longer than 4 counts each time. Concentrate on the exhalation, totally emptying your lungs progressively with each exhalation by pulling in your abdominal muscles.

1. Lie on the floor on your back with your arms at your sides, palms facing up, feet flopped apart.
2. Squeeze your shoulder blades together to open up your chest.
3. Watch your breath, in and out, for 3 breaths. Begin to slow your breathing.
4. Inhale slowly as you count to 4, then exhale for 4 counts by contracting your abdomen.
5. Inhale as you count to 4, then exhale as you count to 5.
6. Continue inhaling for 4 and increasing the length of the exhalation by 1 count each time until you are exhaling for 10 counts.
7. Release by taking a Full Yoga Breath (see Breathe on page 68 for detailed instructions), and relax.
8. Repeat, starting with 4-count inhalations and 4-count exhalations, increasing the length of the exhalation by 1 count each time until you are exhaling for 10 counts.
9. Return to your own breathing pattern, and relax. Notice how clean your lungs feel and how easy it is to breathe. Become aware of any sensations in your body after completing this technique, and enjoy a few moments of stillness as a result of your mind slowing down.

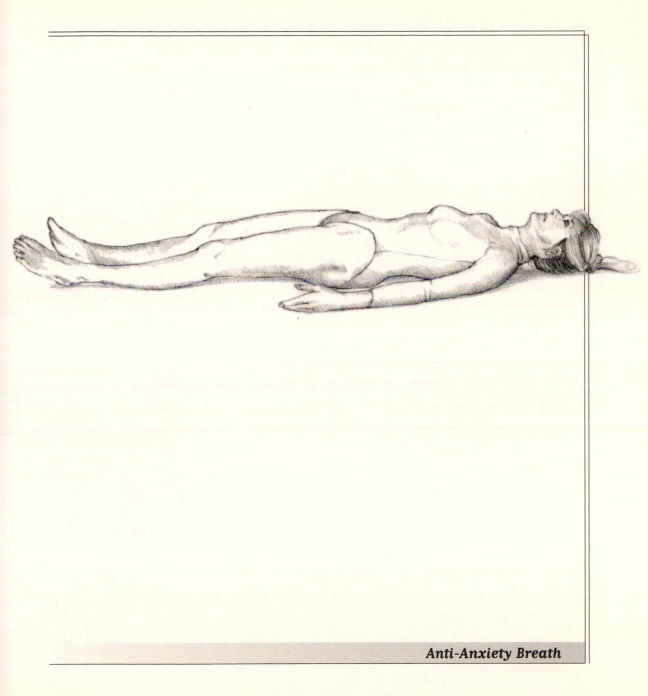

VISUALIZE

A Visit to a Wise Old Woman

This visualization allows you to access your deep, intuitive wisdom that knows the answers to all questions about your health. You only need to create the right conditions for this to occur by practicing a relaxing breathing technique that quiets your mind. In this quiet, reflective state, you can ask a question, sit quietly, then expect to "hear" the answer.

Benefits

Develops intuitive wisdom for self-healing

Focus

Make the lengths of your inhalations, exhalations, and holding of your breath the same.

1. Sit on the floor in Cross-Legged Position. (**Note:** If this position is not comfortable, sit on a folded towel to tilt your hips forward and take the pressure off your knees. Alternatively, sit with your legs stretched out in front, leaning against a wall if necessary, or sit in a chair.)

2. Close your eyes. Begin to observe your breath in a very detached way.

3. Inhale for a count of 4, hold your breath for a count of 4, exhale for a count of 4, and hold your breath for a count of 4. (This is one round.) Complete 7 rounds of this breathing technique as you become as still as a statue.

4. Imagine that you are walking along a beach. You see a path in the sand dunes that leads to an old house.

5. You walk up the path and come to a door with carved symbols on the door. As you look at the door, it opens.

6. You step inside into a long passage lined with books.

7. You walk along this passage until you come to a room where a wise old woman is sitting at a desk.

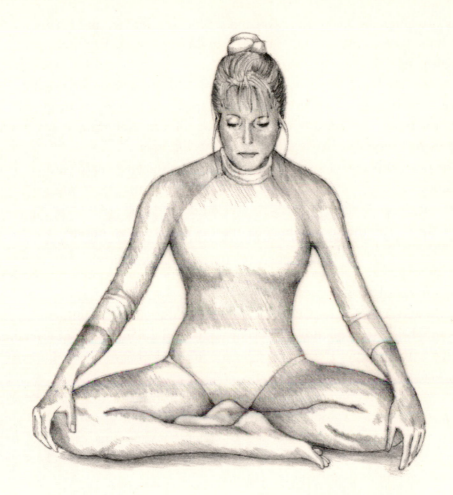

Cross-Legged Position

A Visit to a Wise Old Woman

8. As you enter, she looks up at you and smiles. See her face and her eyes. Ask the wise woman "What do I need to do to enjoy perfect health and well-being?"

9. The woman hands you a dark purple book with your name engraved on the cover in gold; you take the book and sit at a large desk. In this book are the universal records of everything that you are, everything that you can be—and everything that you will be in this lifetime.

10. The book falls open to a page on which appear the answers to your question.

11. Sit quietly, and reflect on what you see on these pages.

12. See the images that appear in your mind of how you can improve your health.

13. Sit quietly in the silence. Watch your breath, your posture, and the images in your mind in a very detached way.

14. In the silence, listen to your own interior world for 10–15 minutes.

15. Gently bring your mind back to your body on the floor and your awareness back to the present. Deepen your breath, and welcome it as your life force and energy source.

16. Let your chin fall to your chest, then drop your head backward to stretch through your neck. Rotate your neck a few times, then sit quietly. You are now ready to get on with your day, knowing that those images of how to improve your health have been firmly imprinted on your subconscious mind and are ready for you to actualize.

A Visit to a Wise Old Woman

chapter seven

Routine 4

Routine 4 builds strength and tone in the thighs and calves to create long, lean muscles. The thighs are the largest muscles in the body. Increasing the percentage of lean muscle in your legs will greatly improve your body's overall metabolic rate to burn fat in the difficult areas (i.e., abdomen, hips, and thighs). The poses convey several benefits:

➤ **Floor Lunge** deeply stretches and tones your hamstrings.

➤ **Balanced Toe Stretch** improves the strength and tone of your abdominal and back muscles for improved posture and balance.

➤ **Liver-Stimulating Exercise** improves the vitality of your liver.

➤ **Vinyasa 4** strengthens and tones all the muscles and joints of your legs. It also strengthens and improves the flexibility of your wrists.

➤ **Lung Expansion Breath** improves the strength of your pectoral muscles to deepen your breath and improve your respiration and combustion rates to metabolize food. It also releases neck and shoulder tension.

➤ **Uncluttering the Mind** is a visualization that shows you how unimportant and useless most of your daily thinking is and teaches you to detach from those thoughts. You then can free up your energy and focus on the more important self-motivational and inspirational thoughts that will help you reach your lifestyle goals.

Did You Know?

To lose weight during menopause, you need to exercise a lot more to increase your metabolic rate. Yoga is the perfect activity because it is so enjoyable, it motivates you to stay active. It also balances the hormone levels that can go a bit haywire during menopause.

STRETCH AND TONE

Floor Lunge

Benefits

Builds upper-arm strength; strongly stretches the hamstrings

Focus

Straighten your leg as much as possible and feel the deep stretch in your inner thighs.

1. Kneel on the floor. Step your right foot forward into a lunge. Place both hands on your right knee, one on top of the other. Rock back and forth 3 times to warm up your knees.

2. Clasp your hands together, and make a triangle with your elbows. Place your elbows on the floor, inside your right foot. Turn the toes of your left foot under.

3. Inhaling, straighten your left leg behind you. Exhaling, bend your left leg so it rests back on floor. Repeat the bending-and-straightening movement 3 times, then lower your knee to the floor.

4. Ease your hands back up onto your right knee, and lunge back and forth 3 times.

5. Step your right leg back to a kneeling position.

6. Step your left foot forward into a lunge. Repeat the sequence 3 times by first rocking back and forth, then bending and straightening the right leg.

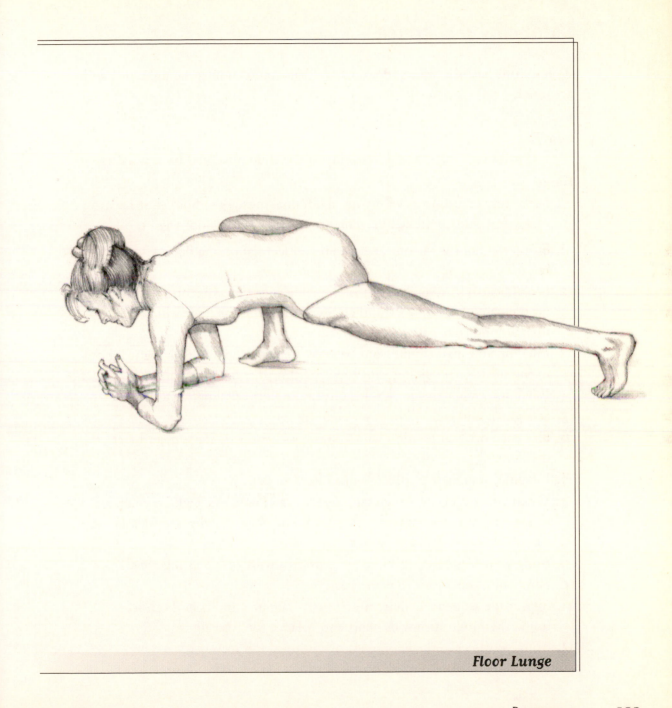

Floor Lunge

IMPROVE POSTURE

Balancing Toe Stretch

To hold this balance, your abdominal and back muscles must be tightened and activated.

Benefits

Improves the strength and flexibility of the abdominal and back muscles

Focus

Make tiny adjustments with your abdominal muscles to hold your balance; make slow and controlled movements when widening your legs.

1. Sit on the floor with your knees bent and feet flat on the floor. Clasp both big toes, and rest your elbows inside your knees.

2. Lean back so that your weight is evenly balanced on your sitting bones (at the base of the buttocks), then lift both feet of the floor while maintaining your balance.

3. Inhaling and maintaining your balance, slowly straighten your right leg out to the side. Keep holding your toes! Exhaling, bend your right knee.

4. Inhaling, straighten your left leg out to the side; exhaling, bend it.

5. Straighten and bend 7 times on each side.

6. Sit in the original position with your knees bent, toes clasped, and feet off the floor.

7. Inhaling, straighten both legs out in front of you.

8. When you are steady, widen your legs as far as possible. Tighten your abdominal muscles. Hold the pose for 3 Full Yoga Breaths (see Breathe on page 68 for detailed instructions).

9. Bring your legs together. Hold for 3 breaths with your legs together.

10. Bend your knees back to your chest.

11. Repeat the sequence 2 more times: first straighten and bend both legs 7 times, then pull them wide apart and balance for 3 breaths.

12. Bring your feet to the floor, release your toes, and relax.

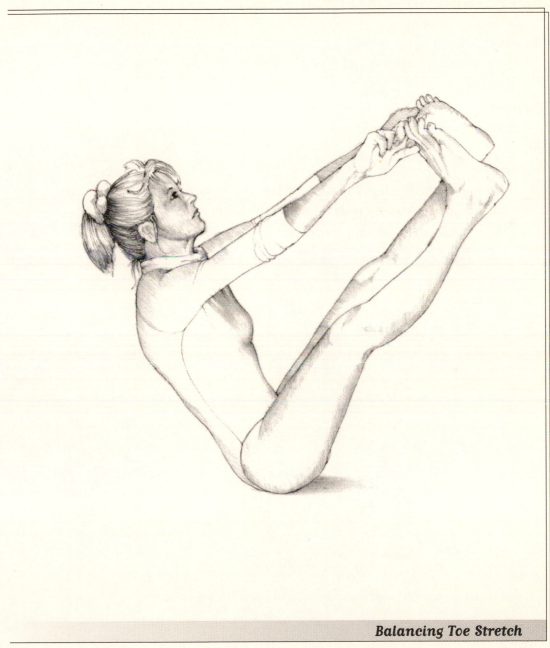

Balancing Toe Stretch

IMPROVE DIGESTION AND ELIMINATION

Liver-Stimulating Exercise

Benefits

Increases the circulation and flow of prana to the liver to improve its function

Focus

Firmly massage your abdomen.

STAGE 1

1. Stand with your feet hip-width part. Place the palm of your right hand on your right upper abdomen, at the base of your rib cage.

Step 1

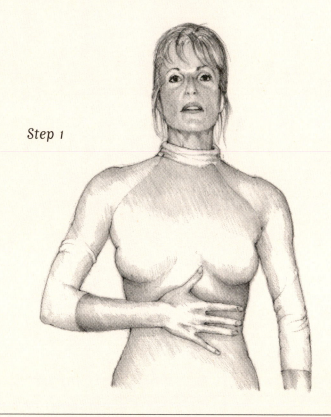

STAGE 2

2. Press your palm across the middle of your abdomen along your lower rib bones.

3. Push your palm up to your breastbone, to the left about 6 inches, down your lower rib bones, and back across to the right lower rib bones. (This pushing from right to left and back again constitutes one repetition.)

4. Repeat this movement firmly 36 times.

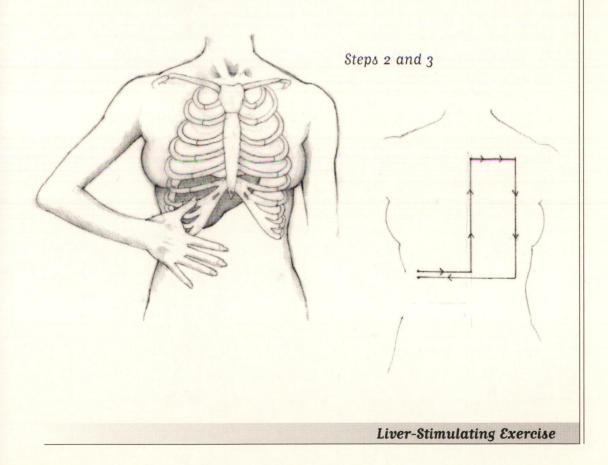

Steps 2 and 3

Liver-Stimulating Exercise

IMPROVE METABOLIC RATE

Vinyasa 4

The repeated jumping in this sequence is an energetic way to build muscle in your legs. It will increase your heart rate as you move back and forth rapidly while balancing on your wrists.

Benefits

Strengthens leg muscles; prevents stiffness and pain in wrists and ankles by improving circulation

Focus

Jump your feet no more than hip-width apart; turn both feet out so that you can lunge correctly and stay balanced.

1. Stand with your feet hip-width apart. Bring your hands to the front of your chest, fingertips together and palms facing down.

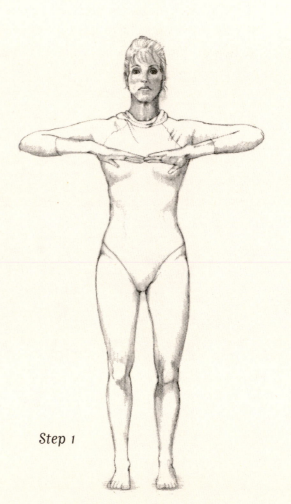

Step 1

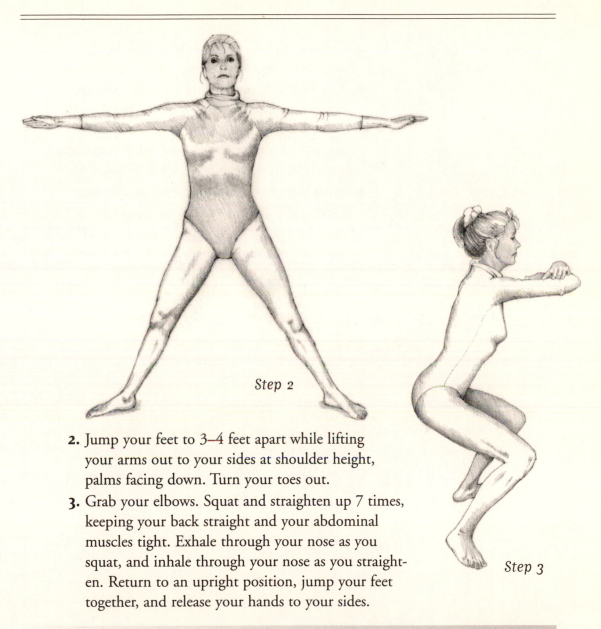

Step 2

Step 3

2. Jump your feet to 3–4 feet apart while lifting your arms out to your sides at shoulder height, palms facing down. Turn your toes out.

3. Grab your elbows. Squat and straighten up 7 times, keeping your back straight and your abdominal muscles tight. Exhale through your nose as you squat, and inhale through your nose as you straighten. Return to an upright position, jump your feet together, and release your hands to your sides.

Vinyasa 4

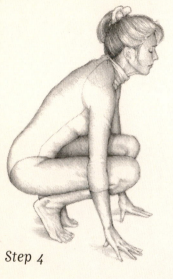

Step 4

4. Squat and place your palms flat on the floor on either side of your feet.

5. Keeping your arms strong and feet together, jump your feet backward and forward 7 times rapidly. Exhale through your nose as you jump your feet backward, and inhale through your nose as you jump your feet forward.

6. Jump your feet backward to hip-width apart. Press into your feet and hands, drop your head between your shoulders, and lift your hips into a strong inverted "V" shape. Bring your weight onto the backs of your heels to press them toward the floor.

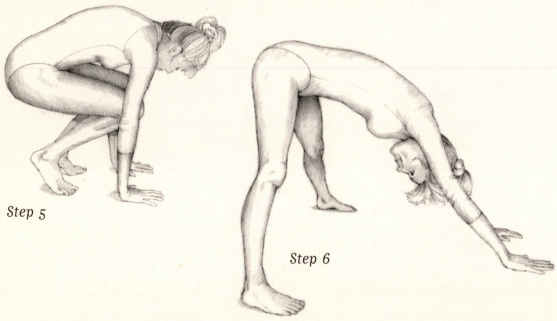

Step 5

Step 6

7. Jump your feet together, "walk" your hands back toward your feet, and squat.

8. Straighten your legs and stand upright. Bring your hands to your chest, fingertips together and palms facing down.

9. Repeat the sequence 3 times, but build up to 7 repetitions over time for maximum benefit.

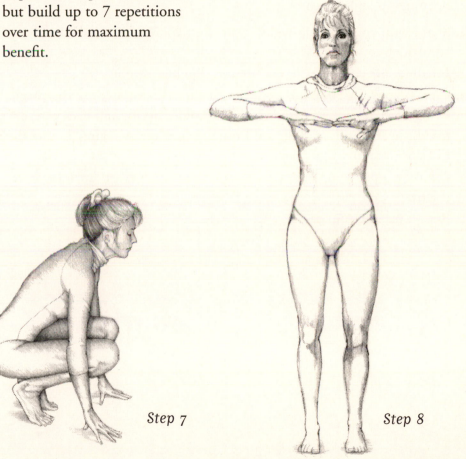

Step 7

Step 8

Vinyasa 4

BREATHE

Lung Expansion Breath

Benefits

Releases tension and stiffness in the neck and shoulders; increases oxygen levels in the blood; increases metabolic rate

Focus

Pull your arms back quite vigorously as you feel your pectoral muscles opening up and stretching.

1. Stand with your legs hip-width apart. Rest your palms on the fronts of your thighs.
2. Inhaling, lift your arms to the front at shoulder height.
3. Clench your fists. Holding your breath and without arching your back, swing both arms out to your sides at shoulder height and back to the middle again. Still holding your breath, repeat the swinging 6 more times. (This is one round.)
4. Exhaling, open your hands and release your palms back down to your thighs.
5. Repeat 6 more rounds.

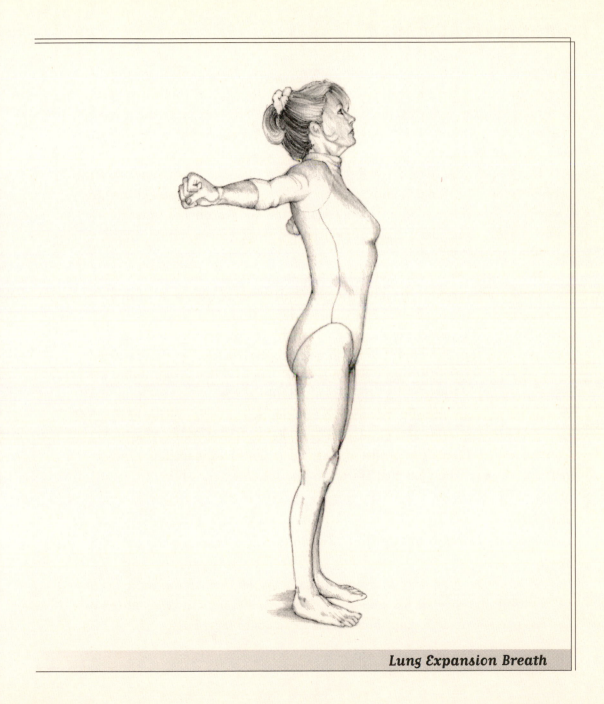

Lung Expansion Breath

VISUALIZE

Uncluttering the Mind

We spend much of our day thinking—escaping into daydreams, worrying about the past, and never fully living in the present. We may think that we are planning, solving problems, or creating new ideas, but most often the mind is merely talking to itself. It is a way of escaping the responsibility of dealing with everyday problems.

This visualization exercise will show you how much of your day is taken up with unimportant thinking and help you to detach from the useless thoughts. Dozens of thoughts can occur in only 5 minutes, and learning to quiet them can take years of regular practice. Practice the art of patience simultaneously with the art of detachment!

As you quiet the mind, you will be able to go beneath this mental clutter and make contact with your subconscious. This is where your state of inner calm exists and where all your motivational, inspirational, and intuitive thoughts lie. You then can get in touch with the limitless ability and intelligence of your mind and body. You will begin to see how they can work together to create perfect health and well-being. The onus and the responsibility are on you; there can be no more blaming others for the shape you are in physically, mentally, or emotionally. You must create the right conditions for healing to occur within your body and mind. You can take control of your eating and exercise program for life by realizing that you are far more than the unimportant and negative thoughts that appear to be controlling your life.

Benefits

Promotes calmness and overall well-being

Focus

As you relax, do not try to stop your thoughts; let them come and go. Tell yourself that they are not important right now. Do not criticize yourself or become frustrated if your mind seems to be continually busy.

PART 1

Chair Position

1. Take a pen and pencil, and have a watch or clock nearby.

2. Sit on the floor in Cross-Legged Position, with your spine straight. (**Note:** If this position is not comfortable, sit on a folded towel to tilt your hips forward and take the pressure off your knees. Alternatively, sit with your legs stretched out in front, leaning against a wall if necessary, or sit in a chair.) Soften your shoulder blades and the muscles around your mouth. Let the tip of your tongue rest gently against the roof of your mouth right behind your teeth to help your jaw and mouth to relax.

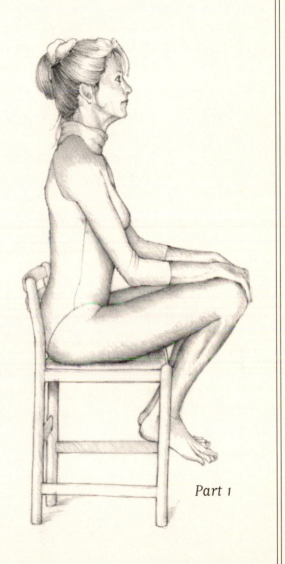

Part 1

Chair Position

3. After several breaths, begin to become aware of your breath. Observe your breath settling into its normal breathing pattern.

4. Notice the thoughts coming into your consciousness. Write down each and every thought that comes into your mind for 5 minutes.

5. Look back over your list and ask yourself the following questions:

➤ How many of these thoughts have to do with planning, solving problems, or creating new ideas?

➤ How many of these thoughts are just conversations with myself; criticisms or comments about others, or fears about the past or future?

PART 2

Relaxed Pose

6. Lie on the floor on your back with your arms at your sides, palms facing up, and feet flopped apart.

7. Return your attention to your breathing. On the inhalation, let your abdomen balloon out a little and be very soft. On the exhalation, consciously pull your abdomen back in. Let the inhalation be soft and expansive, whereas the exhalation is firm and contracting. Continue breathing like this for 20 breaths, then rest briefly in your normal breathing pattern. (This is one round.)

8. Practice attention to your breathing this way for 1 more round, then relax and lie quietly, allowing your mind to settle.

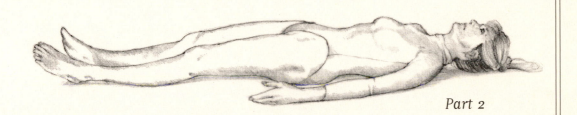

Part 2

9. Repeat the following statements to yourself 3 times:

> I am not my thoughts.
> I am not my body.
> I am not my emotions.
> I am far greater than the sum of all of these.
> For I am pure consciousness.
> I am pure intuitive wisdom—a wisdom that knows
> how to heal my body of any imbalances.

10. Be as still as a statue as you observe your breathing. Listen in the silence of the meditation to what your body and mind are telling you.

11. Lie in the silence for approximately 15 minutes.

12. When you are ready, gently bring yourself back to the present by increasing the depth of your breathing, then stretching your arms overhead a few times.

Relaxed Pose

chapter eight

Routine 5

Routine 5 improves the strength and flexibility of your wrists, shoulders, and ankles to confidently support your weight and to build long, lean muscles and strong bones. The poses convey several benefits:

➤ **Steepled Shoulder Squeeze** fully rotates your wrists and shoulders and improves focus and concentration.

➤ **Half Boat** strengthens and tones your lower-back muscles to improve your posture.

➤ **Stimulating the Kidneys** energizes your kidneys, which are one of the main filters of the body. Kidneys are responsible for eliminating the body's toxins and for maintaining the proper alkaline/acid balance in the body. It also stimulates your adrenal glands to reduce stress levels.

➤ **Vinyasa 5** improves the strength and flexibility of your abdominal muscles and hips.

Did You Know?

Your mind controls where your fat is stored. Research shows that the increase in the stress hormone cortisol, coupled with adrenaline during times of stress, can drive fat into the abdomen. It seems that stress actually causes our bodies to redistribute fat from the thighs to the abdomen, the danger zone that is associated with an increased risk of heart disease. The practice of yoga helps you deal with physical, mental, and emotional stress and lowers your chances of storing excess fat in the abdomen.

➤ **Bellows Breath** cleanses your body of toxins. It also strengthens and tones your abdominal muscles so that you have a stronger eliminatory system as well as a flatter abdomen.

➤ **Mental Housekeeping** is a visualization that clears your mind of mental clutter and improves the quality of your sleep. When you consciously let go of mental clutter before sleeping, you will awake to feel refreshed, renewed, and ready for the day ahead, with all of your body systems energized. When it's combined with soothing music or a warm bath before bedtime, this visualization promotes a deep, relaxing, and restorative sleep.

STRETCH AND TONE

Steepled Shoulder Squeeze

Benefits

Improves flexibility of the wrists and shoulders; stretches hamstrings; gives the heart a rest

Focus

Keep both legs straight, and press your palms together firmly.

1. Stand with your feet 4–6 feet apart, toes turned out slightly.
2. Raise your arms to shoulder height, then bend them and take them behind your back. Bring your fingertips together, palms resting on your lower back.
3. Rotate your wrists so that your palms face out (backs of your hands against your back), fingertips still together. Lean forward, and drop your head down so that it is lower than your heart.
4. Press your fingers up along your spine, toward your shoulder blades. At the same time, ease your palms toward each other, fingers pointing toward your head. The pull of gravity will help you bring your palms closer and higher between your shoulder blades. Pull your shoulders back, and bring your palms together firmly.
5. Turn your left foot in slightly. Inhaling, bring your upper body over your right leg. Exhaling, lower your head toward your knee.
6. Inhaling and exhaling through your nose deeply and slowly, hold the pose for 3 Full Yoga Breaths (see Breathe on page 68 for detailed instructions). On each exhalation, lengthen your body down along your thigh.
7. Inhaling, slowly bring your upper body back to the center.
8. Turn your left foot out and your right foot in slightly. Inhaling, bring your upper body over your left leg. Exhaling, lower your head over your left knee. Hold the pose for 3 Full Yoga Breaths. Focus on lengthening your upper body with each exhalation.
9. Inhaling, bring your body back to the center, and slowly return to an upright position. Breathe normally.

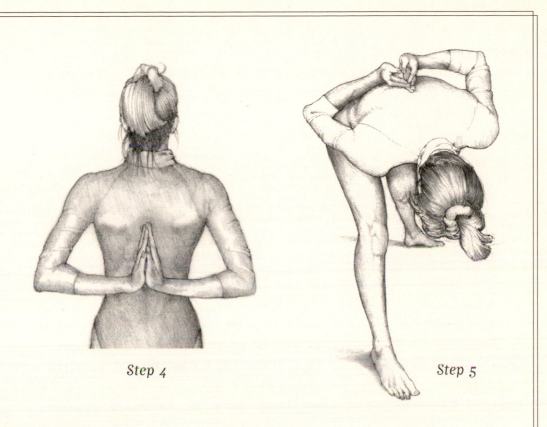

Step 4

Step 5

10. Very gently, release your hands and flick your wrists strongly (as if you have something sticky on your fingers) to release any stiffness in your wrists.

(**Note:** Be very gentle with your body in this pose; do not try to force your palms together. Move with awareness as you bring your body to each side, so there is no strain on your rib muscles.)

Steepled Shoulder Squeeze

IMPROVE POSTURE

Half Boat

Benefits

    Improves the strength and flexibility of the muscles that support the spine; improves posture (giving a slimmer appearance) by strengthening back and abdominal muscles

Focus

    Straighten and lengthen your spine to minimize strain on your lower back. Pull up through your breastbone; do not collapse the chest, because this action will put pressure on your lower-back muscles. Let your abdominal muscles be soft, and focus on using your inner thighs to hold the pose.

    Warning: If you experience chronic back pain or have injured your back, consult an experienced yoga instructor before practicing this pose.

1. Sit on the floor with your legs extended in front of you.
2. Lift and lengthen through your spine, and clasp your hands behind your head, elbows back.
3. Tighten your abdominal muscles, then lean back onto your sitting bones while lifting both feet off the floor a few inches. Extend through your legs, and point your toes. Pull your elbows backward.
4. Breathe deeply through your nose. Hold the pose steady for 3 breaths.
5. Lower your feet and hands to the floor.
6. Bend forward toward your toes, and stretch through your spine.
7. Repeat the pose a total of 3 times; over time, aim to hold the pose for 7 breaths.

(**Note:** If your abdominal muscles are weak and you find that it is too much strain to lift your legs off the floor, begin by bending your knees and lifting your feet off the floor, then straightening your legs.)

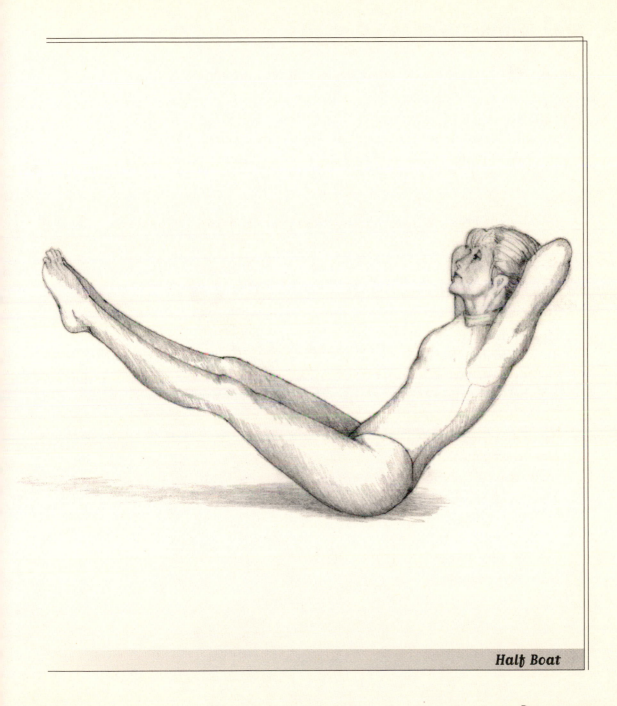

Half Boat

IMPROVE DIGESTION AND ELIMINATION

Stimulating the Kidneys

This simple Chinese exercise should be done in the morning.

Benefits

Stimulates the adrenal glands and the kidneys by increasing circulation and the flow of prana; improves eyesight; keeps the skin smooth; strengthens libido

Focus

Imagine the heat and energy flowing from your hands into your kidneys to promote healing.

Kidney Massage

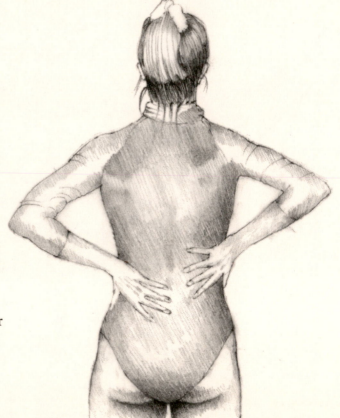

1. Stand with your feet hip-width apart, and lean forward a little. Rub the palms of your hands vigorously together to bring warmth into your hands and fingers, then place your hands over the small of your back.

2. Massage the small of your back by rubbing up and down, then in a circular motion around your lower back for 1 minute.

Pummel Kidneys

3. Clench your fists, and pummel the small of your back for approximately 1 minute.

4. Repeat this alternating massaging and pummeling action for 1 minute at a time until you have completed 5 minutes, total, of both movements.

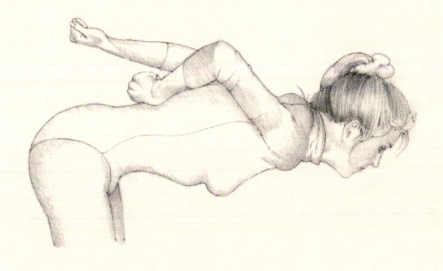

Stimulating the Kidneys

IMPROVE METABOLIC RATE

Vinyasa 5

Vinyasa 5 requires you to lift and lower your legs and to support your body weight on one arm at a time, which strongly activates and tones the deep abdominal muscles for a flatter stomach.

Benefits
Strengthens and tones the abdominal and lower-back muscles; strengthens the muscles and bones in the upper arms; builds confidence in your ability to support and balance your weight for short periods

Focus
Feel light as you lift your body off the floor and strong as you balance. When taking your legs sideways to the floor, keep pressing your lower back into the floor as you lower your legs to protect your lower back. Do not hold your breath while lowering your legs, because this creates tension in your abdominal muscles. Keep your breath smooth and rhythmic to avoid jarring the muscles of your back or groin. When lowering both legs to the floor, aim to keep them level with your outstretched arms.

1. Lie on the floor on your back, bend your knees, and take hold of your ankles. Place your feet on the floor beside your buttocks. Release your hands to the floor, arms stretched out at shoulder height, palms facing down.

2. Inhale deeply. Exhaling, lower both knees to the right while turning your head to the left and pressing your left shoulder down. Press your left knee closer to the floor to increase the stretch in your hip. Return to center. Lower both legs to the left while turning your head to the right and pressing your right shoulder down. Repeat 2 more times on each side.

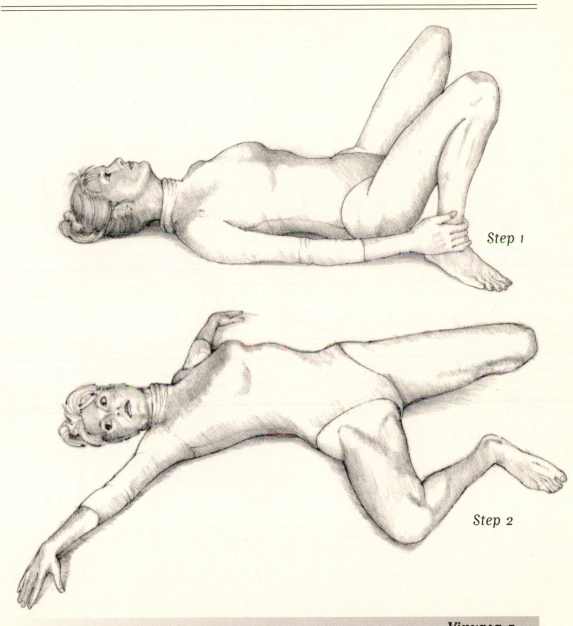

Step 1

Step 2

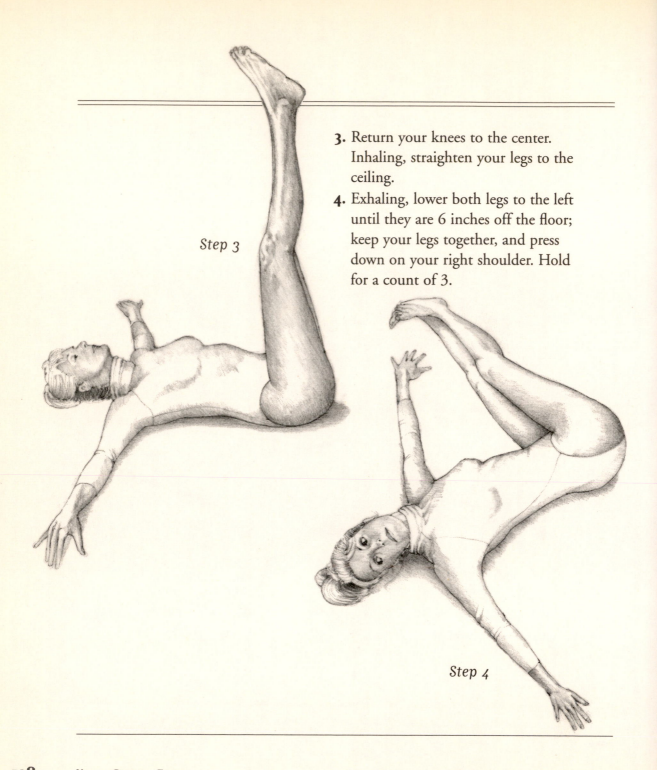

3. Return your knees to the center. Inhaling, straighten your legs to the ceiling.

4. Exhaling, lower both legs to the left until they are 6 inches off the floor; keep your legs together, and press down on your right shoulder. Hold for a count of 3.

Step 3

Step 4

5. Inhaling, return your legs to the center, legs together. Exhaling, lower both legs to the right until they are 6 inches off the floor; keep your legs together, and press down on your left shoulder. Hold for a count of 3. Repeat the leg lifts 3 times on each side.

6. Bring your legs back to the center, bend your knees, roll onto your left side, and sit up. Straighten your legs out to the side, in line with your hips, and place both palms flat on the floor in front of your hips.

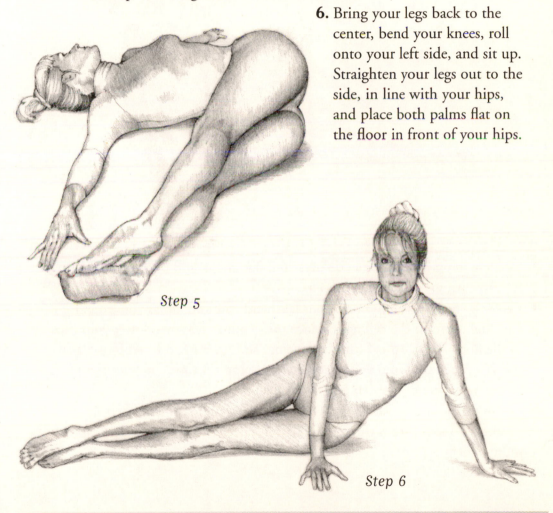

Step 5

Step 6

Vinyasa 5

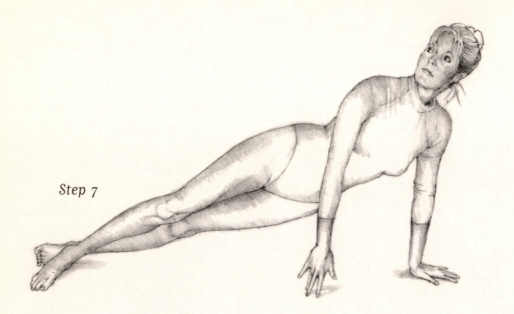

Step 7

7. Inhaling, cross your right ankle over your left ankle, and push on your arms to lift your hips as high as you can.

8. Exhaling, take your weight on your left hand and look up as you extend your right arm to the ceiling. Balance for a count of 3, then lower your hips to the floor. Repeat this lifting, balancing, and lowering 3 times in total on this side, then roll onto your right side and repeat 3 times on your right arm as you extend your left arm to the ceiling.

9. Lie on the floor on your back, bend your knees, and return to Step 1. Practice the sequence 3 times in total; build up to 7 repetitions for maximum benefit.

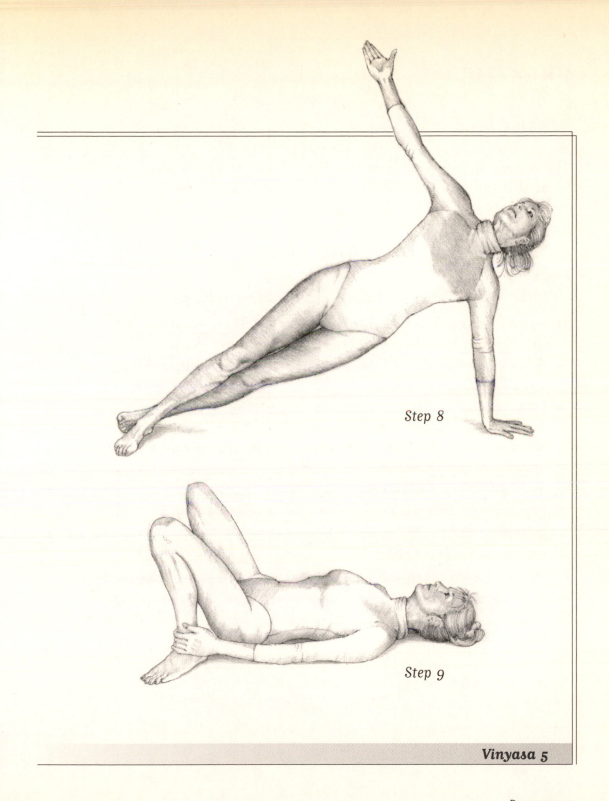

Step 8

Step 9

Vinyasa 5

BREATHE

Bellows Breath

The Bellows Breath is the complete Full Yoga Breath (see Breathe on page 68 for detailed instructions) performed with an accelerated rhythm.

Benefits

Tones all the muscles of the abdomen and chest

Focus

Make your inhalation sudden and your exhalation forceful.

1. Sit back on your heels, and rest your hands loosely on your knees. Lift and lengthen your spine to open up your chest.

2. Inhale and exhale slowly 3 times as you observe your breath settle into your normal breathing pattern.

3. Fill your lungs suddenly and forcefully by breathing in through your nose in the Full Yoga Breath.

4. Without a pause, forcefully exhale through your nose, emptying your lungs by first contracting your abdomen wall, then compressing your ribs, and finally relaxing your shoulders.

5. Repeat the inhalation and exhalation 7 times, then relax and breathe normally.

6. Repeat the inhalation and exhalation again for 7 consecutive breaths.

(**Note:** This is a strong, dynamic breath. If you are not used to breathing deeply you may experience a little lightheadedness. If so, lie down and rest for a few moments. Practice slowly with one sequence before you attempt the second sequence.)

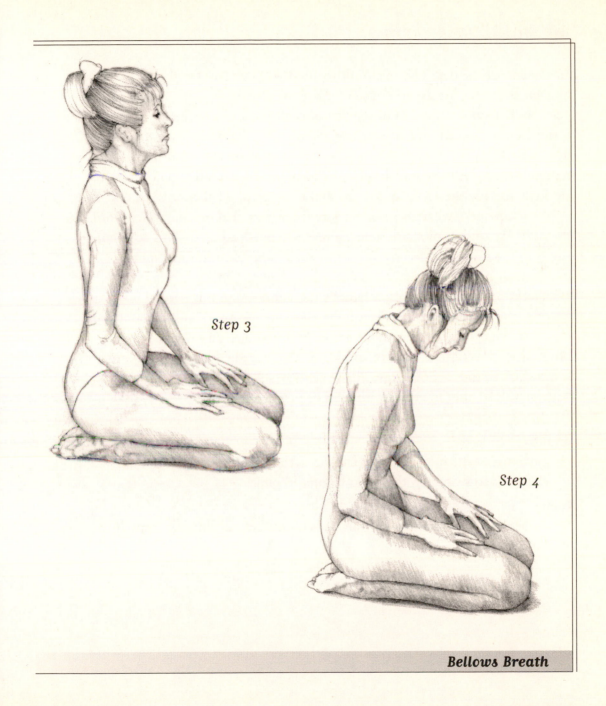

Step 3

Step 4

Bellows Breath

VISUALIZE

Mental Housekeeping

At the end of the day, a normal healthy mind will sort and file things that have happened during the day to prepare for a good night's sleep. It's similar to what goes on in a store at the end of the day, after the doors have closed. Stressors—insufficient or interrupted sleep, chronic tension in the body, illness, or major upheavals (e.g., moving, changing jobs, death, or divorce)—interrupt this natural process. All stressors diminish in some way the mind's ability to sort through and file the events of the day and to let go of what is finished.

Consequently, what does not get sorted out and filed one day is left until the next day, and so on, until it accumulates to overload level. This accumulation can leave a person feeling as if he or she has no room for any more thoughts. It may result in stress, anxiety, and depleted energy levels.

Deep, progressive relaxation retrains the mind to use this natural house-keeping ability by creating a beautifully relaxed body, mind, and emotions so that this work can continue, unhindered, in the stillness. The magic of deep, progressive relaxation is that you awaken with a refreshed mind, body, and spirit—full of focus and energy. The benefits of relaxing the mind deeply can be experienced after even a few minutes of practice.

Benefits

Encourages the mind to relax; enables detachment from unimportant thoughts to switch off the mind before sleeping

Focus

Consciously sort and file all your day's events before allowing yourself to fall asleep.

Relaxed Pose

1. Lie on your bed in Relaxed Pose with arms at your sides, palms facing up, feet flopped apart, and shoulder blades squeezed together to open up your chest. Release the tension in your face by unlocking your jaw and smoothing out your forehead.

2. Observe your breath, and count the length of each inhalation and exhalation. Gradually make your inhalations the same length as your exhalations, pausing for 2 counts after each.

3. Do 7 Full Yoga Breaths (see Breathe on page 68 for detailed instructions), then resume your own breathing pattern.

4. As you observe your breath, feel your body growing lighter and lighter, and allow your thoughts to come and go; they are not important right now. Let any sounds you hear to fade into the distance. Feel a sense of growing detachment from your thoughts.

5. Imagine that you are sitting in a favorite room in a deep comfortable chair in front of a screen, and you have turned on a video of your day's events.

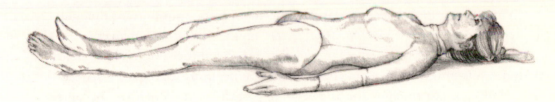

Mental Housekeeping

6. As you watch the video, mentally check off those things that are finished; visualize them being copied from a computer's hard drive (your mind) to a diskette marked "Finished." For things that need to be attended to, make a mental note to look at them tomorrow; visualize yourself placing each item into a paper folder marked "Unfinished."

7. When the video ends, imagine throwing the diskette of "Finished" business into the trash can. Imagine placing the "Unfinished" folder on your bedside table, ready to attend to in the morning.

8. Visualize yourself getting up to draw the curtains in your room. Symbolically draw a curtain across your mind to signify the end of the day, then sink down into that comfortable, deep, velvety darkness behind your eyes.

9. Listen to the silence all around you as you drift down into your own interior world and a deep, relaxing sleep. In the morning, you will remember the imaginary folder beside your bed and all those things you need to do.

10. Practice this technique every night until it becomes automatic and effortless.

(**Note:** If you find that your mind is still full of busy unimportant thoughts after completing this exercise, focus on observing these thoughts in a very detached way, letting them come and go. The more you focus on each thought, the more your mind will become quiet, until you begin to see a space between the end of your last thought and the beginning of the next. When you become aware of that space—that emptiness in your mind—let your mind rest in that space for a moment. You then will be able to drift off to sleep.)

Mental Housekeeping

chapter nine

Routine 6

Routine 6 improves hip and shoulder mobility and increases muscle tone in your thighs and upper arms. The poses convey several benefits:

➤ **Hip Rotation** fully opens your hips so that you can move more easily in and out of yoga poses and can sit comfortably in Cross-Legged Position.

➤ **Full Boat** activates your abdominal muscles deep in your groin and improves balance and concentration.

➤ **Supine Bandha** alerts you to any sore spots in your abdomen, which may be signs of constipation.

➤ **Vinyasa 6** is a strong and empowering sequence that works on every major joint in your body. It also builds balance, and the more you practice, the more confident you become in moving from one pose to the next. That feeling of physical balance carries over into feelings of mental and emotional balance to promote inner harmony and feeling good about yourself.

➤ **Hissing Cobra** helps to clear out stale, heavy air from deep within your lungs that may be making you feel tired or lethargic. It greatly enhances your immune system by flushing your thymus gland with fresh oxygenated blood when you release the pose.

➤ **A Lake** is a visualization that provides you with a graphic image of how "heavy" negative thoughts can make you feel by linking negative thoughts with the image of heavy mud sinking to the bottom of a lake.

Did You Know?

Small changes can make a big difference to your metabolic rate. For example, taking 7 Full Yoga Breaths (see BREATHE in Chapter 5 for detailed instructions) on awakening every morning increases the oxygen supply to all the cells of your body. As a result, your metabolic rate increases to help combust food and burn calories.

STRETCH AND TONE

Hip Rotation

Benefits

Nourishes and opens up the hips fully; tones the muscles of the waist

Focus

Keep your legs strong, so that you feel steady to rotate your hips as widely as you can without upsetting your balance.

1. Stand with your feet hip-width apart. Inhaling, circle your arms overhead, and bring your palms together. Interlock your fingers, with index fingers pointing up.

2. Look up at your hands. With your pointed fingers, "draw" a small, imaginary circle on the ceiling in a clockwise direction. Move your hips at the same time, also in a clockwise direction.

3. Make a slightly larger circle, with your arm and hip movements still coordinated.

4. Make progressively larger circles until you have completed 7 circles. With each rotation, stretch and lengthen through your arms and fingers as you bend forward, sideways, and backward. Bend fully in each direction until you feel your waist and back muscles begin to work. On the last rotation, your interlocked fingers should come low to the floor as you bend forward.

5. Pause and rest.

6. Start "drawing" large circles, close to the ground, in a counterclockwise direction. Make progressively smaller circles as you come back to the starting position, with your arms directly above your head.

7. Repeat the sequence in reverse, starting with small counterclockwise circles that get progressively larger, then making large clockwise circles that get progressively smaller.

8. Drop your arms to your sides, shrug your shoulders, and relax.

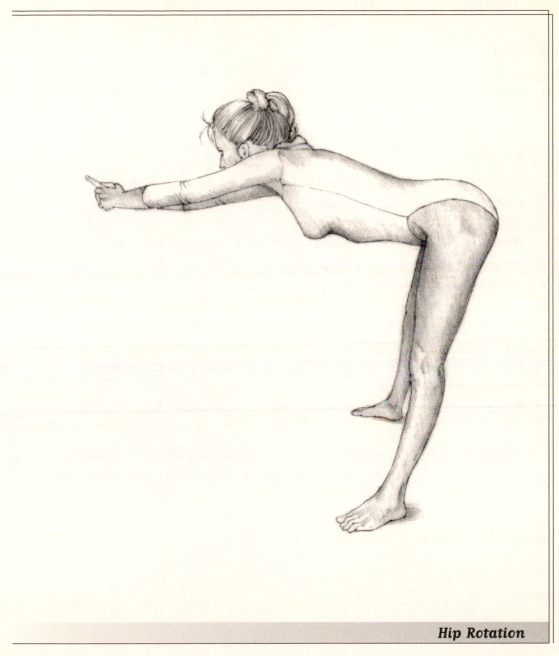

Hip Rotation

IMPROVE POSTURE

Full Boat

Benefits

Improves the strength and flexibility of abdominal and back muscles; improves balance and concentration

Focus

Stretch and lengthen through your spine to make your spine very strong, to help lift your legs without straining your lower back.

1. Sit on the floor with your legs extended in front of you. Stretch up through your spine, arching your back slightly. Rest your palms on top of your thighs.

2. Initially, tighten your abdominal muscles, then lean back onto your sitting bones. Lift your feet off the floor a few inches while extending your arms up and forward, toward your feet.

3. Hold your balance, and steady your breath. Relax your abdominal muscles and point your toes. Keep extending through your arms and legs, and breathe deeply for 3 breaths.

4. Lower your feet and hands to the floor. Bend forward toward your toes, and lengthen your spine.

5. Repeat the pose again. Aim to practice 3 times and to hold for 7 breaths each time.

(**Note:** If you feel any strain in your back, release the pose and rest. Yoga is a diagnostic tool; it will show you the weaknesses in your body that need to be strengthened, so do not criticize yourself if you cannot achieve a pose. In time, as you practice all of the poses in this book, your muscles will strengthen, and you will be able to practice this wonderful pose.)

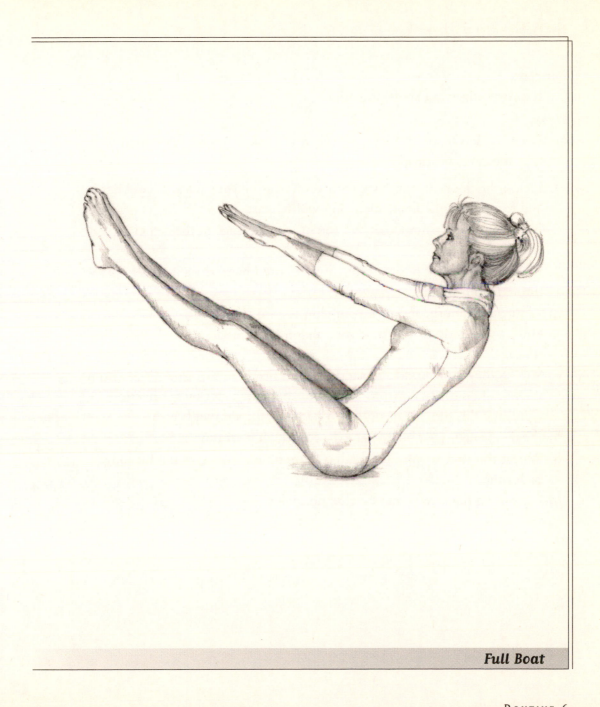

Full Boat

IMPROVE DIGESTION AND ELIMINATION

Supine Bandha

Benefits

Improves digestion and elimination

Focus

Pay attention to any tender spots when you massage your abdomen; they may indicate constipation.

1. Lie on the floor on your back with your arms by your sides, knees bent, and feet flat on the floor, about hip-width apart.

2. Place your right palm loosely on top of your rib cage in the center of your chest.

3. Inhale a deep, slow breath through your nose, then exhale it forcefully through your mouth.

4. Close your mouth, and tuck your chin toward your chest.

5. Hold your breath as you suck your abdominal muscles up and under your rib cage.

6. Still holding your breath, move your palm firmly in big, slow circles from the top of your ribs down to your pubic bone in a clockwise direction. Continue this movement until you need to take another breath.

7. Inhale through your nose, and exhale through your mouth.

8. Repeat the circles with the breath 6 more times, aiming to hold it longer each time.

9. Lay on the floor, relax and breathe normally.

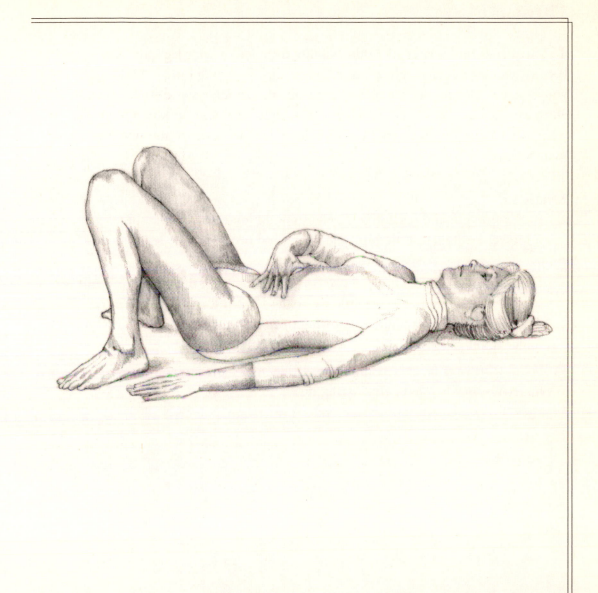

Supine Bandha

IMPROVE METABOLIC RATE

Vinyasa 6

This sequence builds strength and flexibility throughout your legs and hips because you take your weight on one leg at a time in strong lunges. Holding your lunge while arching your back opens up your shoulders and stretches your entire spine. The side twists rotate your hips, shoulders, and neck to a point of resistance to improve flexibility. It creates long, lean muscles to improve your metabolic rate.

Benefits
Builds strength and flexibility in the legs and hips; stretches the spine; improves flexibility in the hips, shoulders, and neck

Focus
Look at a point on the floor as you balance on one leg. Breathe deeply and slowly, so that you become a little sweaty and breathless by the end of the sequence. Feel light and agile, knowing that you are not as "heavy" as you might think you are!

1. Stand with your feet hip-width apart. Bring your hands to your chest, fingertips together and palms facing down.

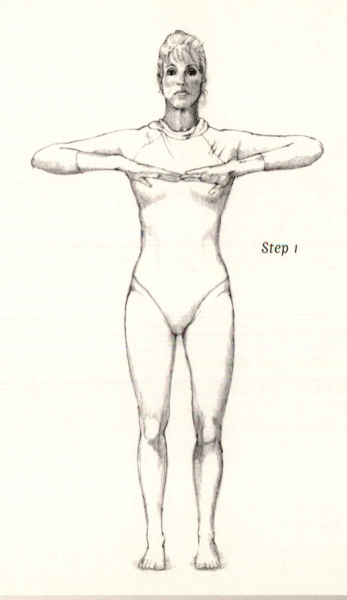

Step 1

Vinyasa 6

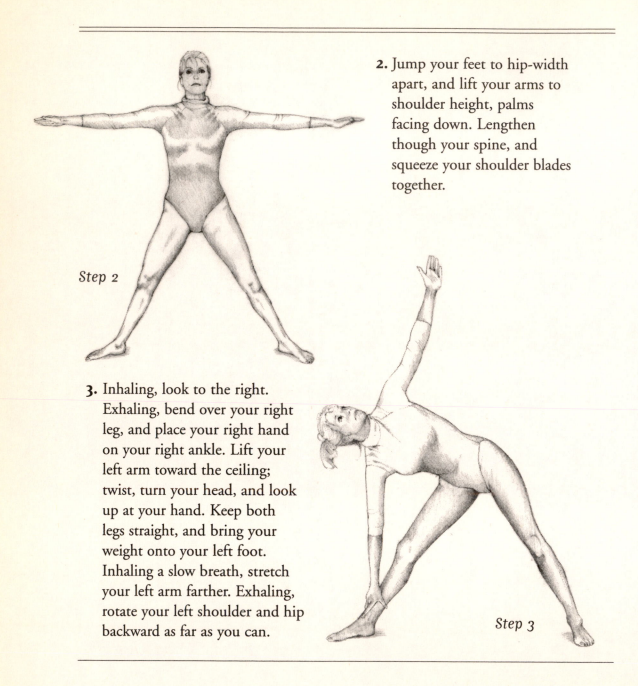

2. Jump your feet to hip-width apart, and lift your arms to shoulder height, palms facing down. Lengthen though your spine, and squeeze your shoulder blades together.

Step 2

3. Inhaling, look to the right. Exhaling, bend over your right leg, and place your right hand on your right ankle. Lift your left arm toward the ceiling; twist, turn your head, and look up at your hand. Keep both legs straight, and bring your weight onto your left foot. Inhaling a slow breath, stretch your left arm farther. Exhaling, rotate your left shoulder and hip backward as far as you can.

Step 3

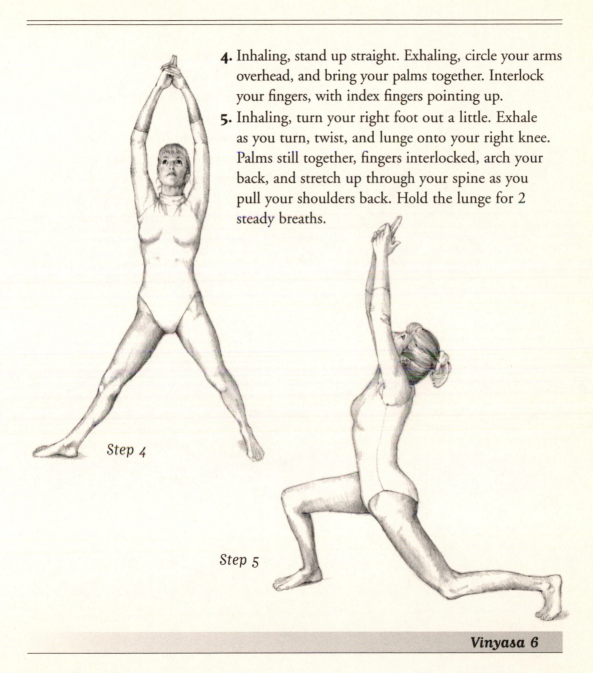

4. Inhaling, stand up straight. Exhaling, circle your arms overhead, and bring your palms together. Interlock your fingers, with index fingers pointing up.

5. Inhaling, turn your right foot out a little. Exhale as you turn, twist, and lunge onto your right knee. Palms still together, fingers interlocked, arch your back, and stretch up through your spine as you pull your shoulders back. Hold the lunge for 2 steady breaths.

Step 4

Step 5

Vinyasa 6

6. Lean forward, and extend your arms to the front so they are parallel to the floor.

7. Slide your left foot in so that you can straighten your right leg. Bring your weight over your right foot. Lock your right knee, lift your left leg straight out behind you, parallel to the floor, lean forward, and stretch your arms forward. Stretch strongly through your legs and arms. Hold the pose steady for 2 breaths.

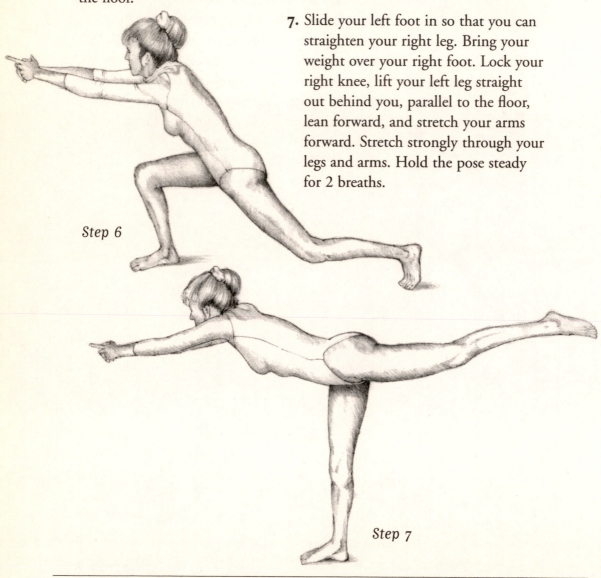

Step 6

Step 7

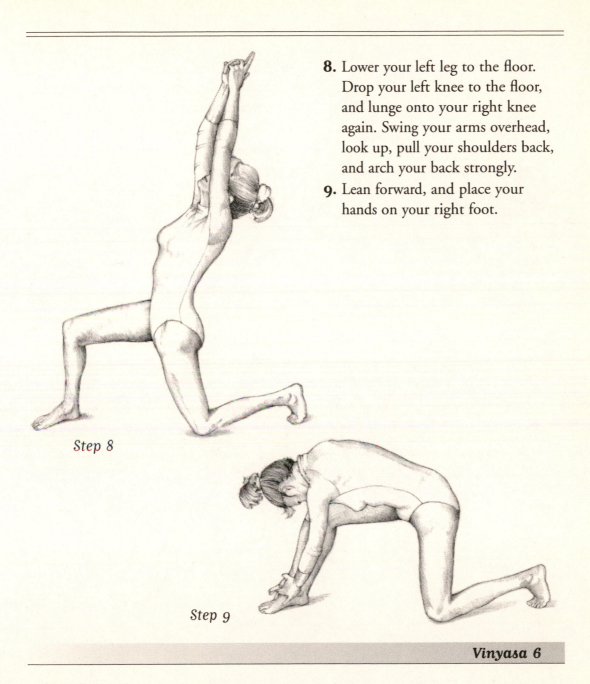

8. Lower your left leg to the floor. Drop your left knee to the floor, and lunge onto your right knee again. Swing your arms overhead, look up, pull your shoulders back, and arch your back strongly.

9. Lean forward, and place your hands on your right foot.

Step 8

Step 9

Vinyasa 6

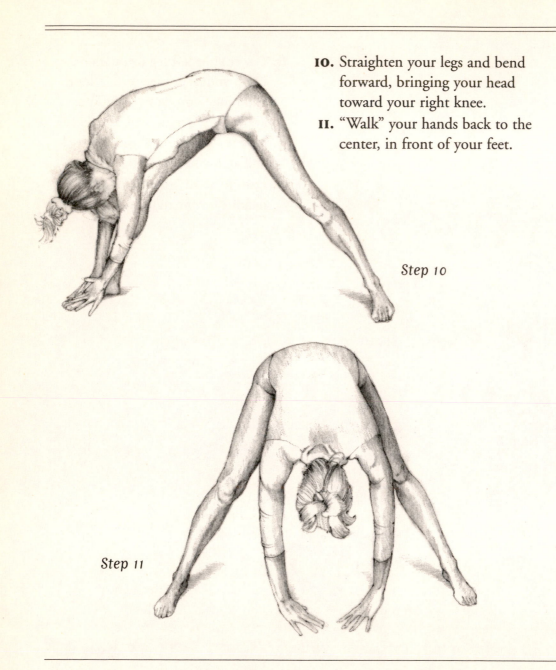

10. Straighten your legs and bend forward, bringing your head toward your right knee.

11. "Walk" your hands back to the center, in front of your feet.

Step 10

Step 11

12. Inhaling, stand up and lift your arms to shoulder height. Exhaling, jump your feet together and your hands to your chest in starting position, fingertips together and palms facing down.

13. Repeat this sequence 7 times while breathing deeply and vigorously. Increase the speed of the sequence as you become familiar with it so that you finish a bit breathless and sweaty.

14. Release your arms to your sides, and relax.

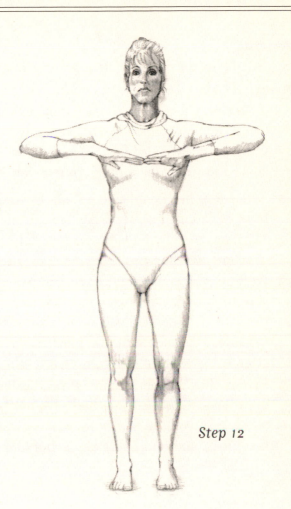

Step 12

Vinyasa 6

BREATHE

Hissing Cobra

Benefits

Forcibly gets rid of stale air and toxins in the bottom of the lungs

Focus

Keep your chest as low to the ground as you can for as long as you can before arching your body. Hiss as loudly as you can for maximum benefit. Once in the extended forward position with your arms locked, keep lengthening and stretching through your abdominal muscles as you hiss.

1. Sit on your heels on the floor. Lean forward and stretch your arms out in front of you, palms flat on the floor. Inhale.

2. Exhaling strongly through your mouth (making a hissing sound), slide your chin and chest forward along the floor. Keep your hips low.

3. Push up with your arms, and support your body on locked elbows; drop your head backward, arch your back, and stretch through your abdomen. Continue hissing until you empty your lungs completely.

4. When you run out of breath, inhale while you sit back on your heels, arms extended in front of you, palms flat on the floor.

5. Repeat Hissing Cobra 6 more times, hissing as you slide forward and inhaling as you sit back on your heels. Do not take any extra breaths in between.

6. Sit back on your heels with your arms outstretched and your head on the floor. Rest, and notice how clean your lungs feel.

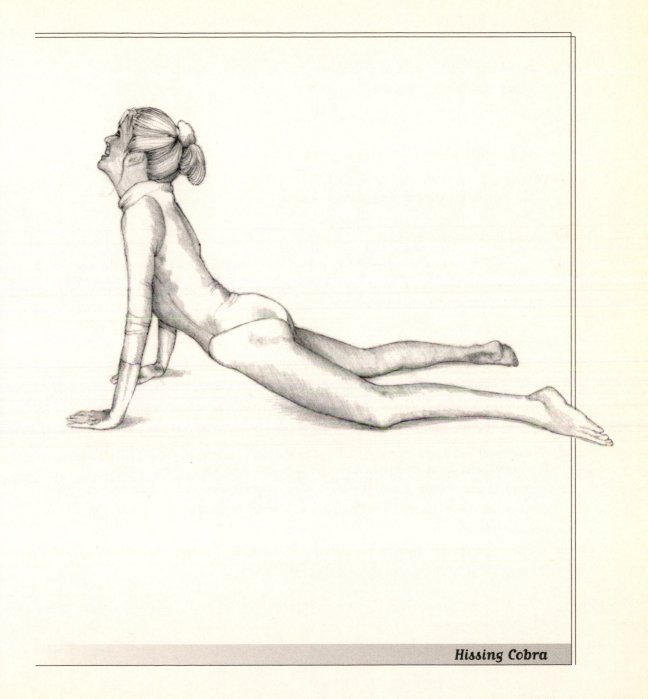

Hissing Cobra

VISUALIZE

A Lake

This visualization creates an uplifting image to raise your spirits. Expect to think more clearly with practice.

Benefits

Enables the release of heavy negative thoughts

Focus

Concentrate on the rhythm of your breath.

Cross-Legged Position

1. Sit on the floor in Cross-Legged Position, with your spine straight and your hands resting lightly on your knees. (**Note:** If this position is not comfortable, sit on a folded towel to tilt your hips forward and take the pressure off your knees. Alternatively, sit with your legs stretched out in front, leaning against a wall if necessary, or sit in a chair.)

2. With your eyes closed, begin to observe your breath. Inhale for a count of 7, hold your breath for 3 counts, exhale for a count of 7, and hold your breath for 3 counts. Repeat the breathing exercise 7 times, then relax and observe the rise and fall of your chest.

3. Imagine that you are sitting beside a beautiful lake. The surface of the lake is smooth like glass, and the sun is shining. See yourself picking up a pebble and throwing it into the lake. Watch the ripples gently disappear. Recognize that negative thoughts have the same rippling effect, disturbing your peace of mind.

4. As you observe the rhythm of your breath, imagine that the natural state of your mind is stillness, like the waters of the lake.

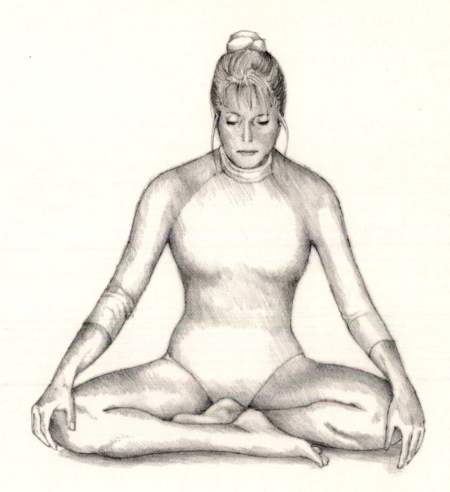

Cross-Legged Position

A Lake

5. Sit quietly, and let your thoughts come and go. Imagine that any negative thoughts in your mind are like mud. If a particular thought disturbs your peace of mind, imagine that thought settling down into the depths of the waters of your mind—like mud sinking to the bottom of a lake—leaving your mind clear and still.

6. Observe your mind settling, bringing clarity to strengthen your focus and concentration.

7. Look deeply into the crystal-clear waters of your mind, and see yourself exactly as you would like to be. As you observe your breath and your thoughts, continue to refine that image of yourself until it is perfect.

8. Hold that perfect image in the silence of the visualization for 10–15 minutes.

9. Take a Full Yoga Breath (see Breathe on page 68 for detailed instructions), and enjoy the sense of stillness that this visualization brings. Throughout the day, practice letting go of thoughts that you do not want: Inhale as you visualize the thoughts as being like mud, then exhale as those thoughts dissolve and sink down to the bottom of the waters of your mind—and stay there.

A Lake

chapter ten

Routine 7

Routine 7 is the most challenging of all the routines presented in this book; it is very strenuous. It should not be practiced until you feel confident with the preceding six routines. The poses convey several benefits:

➤ **Bent-Knee Lunge**, the warm-up stretch, strongly stretches the fronts of your thighs.

➤ **Leg Raises** tone your abdominal and back muscles. The subtle movements of your abdominal muscles while in the balance improve the strength and tone of your back muscles.

➤ **Whipping Bandha** has a wonderful stimulating effect on all of your digestive and eliminatory organs. By improving the function of your pancreas, the bandha balances your sugar and energy levels to avoid highs and lows throughout the day.

➤ **Vinyasa 7** combines your balance, strength, and concentration to build long, lean muscles and increase your metabolic rate. It also improves mind–body awareness and coordination.

➤ **Alternate Nostril Breathing** and **Right Nostril Breathing** are recommended by the 10th International Yoga Therapy Conference for weight loss. The combination improves focus and concentration, calms the nerves, and creates mental stillness and focus.

➤ **Release Old Ideas and Limiting Thoughts** is a visualization that alerts you to any negative thoughts that you are choosing to energize. Practice letting go of negative thoughts and retaining healthy life-sustaining thoughts that will prevent health problems later on in life.

Did You Know?

Regularly practicing yoga will improve your stamina, flexibility, endurance, and concentration in other sports. You will be able to hit a tennis ball harder and a golf ball farther; you will be able to walk for longer distances to burn more calories.

STRETCH AND TONE

Bent-Knee Lunge

Benefits

Increases flexibility in the knees; strengthens the thighs; improves balance and concentration

Focus

Bring all of your weight down through your groin to center and balance your body. Visualize your upper thighs having the stretch of a rubber band, and know that as you breathe and lunge, these muscles will lengthen and grow leaner.

1. Kneel on the floor. Step your right foot forward into a lunge. Keep your left knee on the floor.

2. Place both hands on your right knee, one on top of the other.

3. Inhaling, stretch up through your spine. Exhaling, extend more deeply in the lunge. Bring all of your body weight down through the center of your groin area.

4. Inhaling, return to the relaxed lunge position.

5. Repeat the slow back-and-forth lunge 3 times, stretching more deeply with each lunge to stretch the backs of your thighs. On the last repetition, hold the extended lunge for 7 Full Yoga Breaths (see Breathe on page 68 for detailed instructions). Relax your shoulders.

6. Bend your left heel up to your left buttock, and reach around with your left hand to clasp the top of your left foot firmly.

7. Steady yourself, then reach around with your right hand to clasp the top of your left foot, so that both hands are clasping the front of your left foot. Press your right foot into the floor for balance.

8. Exhaling, lunge more deeply, and pull your left foot closer to your buttocks. Pull slowly, so there is a deep stretch but no strain on the thigh. Inhaling, release your foot away from your buttocks slightly; exhaling, pull it in again. Repeat the lunge-and-pull motion 3 more times.

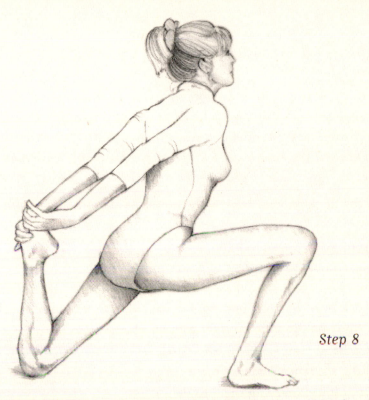

Step 8

9. Release your left foot, and step your right foot back to a kneeling position.

10. Step your left foot forward into a lunge. Place both hands on your left knee, one on top of the other. Repeat the sequence on this side with slow breathing: the back-and-forth lunge 4 times, then the lunge-and-pull motion 4 times with your right heel pulled to your right buttock. On the last repetition, hold the lunge with bent leg for 7 breaths.

11. Release your right foot, and step your left foot back to a kneeling position. Sit on the floor with both legs stretched out in front of you, and rub your legs gently.

Bent-Knee Lunge

IMPROVE POSTURE

Leg Raises

Benefits

Strengthens the lower-back and abdominal muscles

Focus

Press your lower back into the floor as you hold your legs off the floor; do not arch your back. Visualize yourself as having a strong, flat abdomen. See your spine straightening and strengthening with each lift.

Warning: If you have lower-back problems, place your fists under your buttocks for this exercise. Release the pose if you feel any discomfort.

1. Lie on the floor on your back with your arms at your sides, palms facing down.

2. Bend your knees to your chest.

3. Inhaling, straighten your legs to the ceiling.

4. Exhaling, lower your straight legs to about 6 inches off the floor. Press your lower back into the floor, and tighten your abdominal muscles. Hold your breath while holding the pose for a count of 7.

5. Inhaling, bend your knees to your chest.

6. Repeat the sequence 3 more times.

7. Bend your knees and hug them to your chest.

8. Release your legs and arms to the floor. Lie on the floor on your back with your arms at your sides, palms facing down.

9. Inhaling, bend your knees to your chest.

10. Exhaling, extend your legs out straight to about 6 inches off the floor.

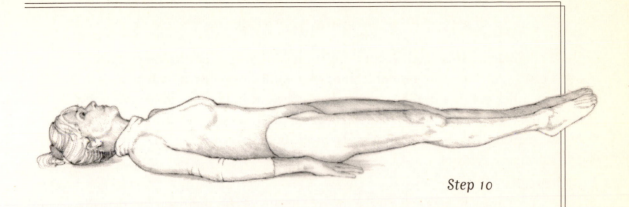

Step 10

11. Press your abdominal and back muscles toward the floor. Hold your breath while holding the pose for a count of 7.
12. Inhaling, raise both straight legs to the ceiling.
13. Exhaling, bend your knees to your chest.
14. Repeat the sequence 3 times.
15. Hug your knees to your chest. Rock backward and forward and from side to side to release any stiffness in your lower back. Let your legs drop to the floor, and relax.

Leg Raises

IMPROVE DIGESTION AND ELIMINATION

Whipping Bandha

Adapted from Lucille Wood, Gita International Yoga Australia, with permission.

If you practice this bandha first thing in the morning after drinking a glass of warm water with a squeeze of lemon, your eliminatory system will be activated very quickly. It is a healthy start to the day before you begin filling your body with food. Its effect on the pancreas (which produces insulin) is to balance sugar levels, and hence energy levels, in the body.

Benefits

Dynamically massages all the internal organs of the abdomen, particularly the pancreas; improves circulation to the abdominal area; nourishes all the organs of digestion to improve their function

Focus

Pull your abdominal muscles up and under your rib cage tightly to create a lock over your pancreas. Watch your abdomen as you practice to get as much movement as possible.

(**Note:** This movement may feel a little awkward until you establish a rhythm. The faster you move your abdomen in and out, the easier it is.)

1. Stand with your legs about 4 feet apart. Bend your knees, and squat with your hands resting on your knees, fingertips facing in.
2. Inhale, then exhale forcefully through your open mouth.
3. Close your mouth, tuck your chin to your chest, and hold your breath.
4. Suck your abdominal muscles back up and under your rib cage.
5. Push your abdomen out strongly first, then move it in and out quickly as you hold your breath. Continue until you run out of breath.
6. Inhaling, straighten your legs.
7. Exhaling, bend forward. Hang loosely. (This completes one repetition.)
8. Repeat the sequence 2 more times, gradually building up to 7 repetitions per day.

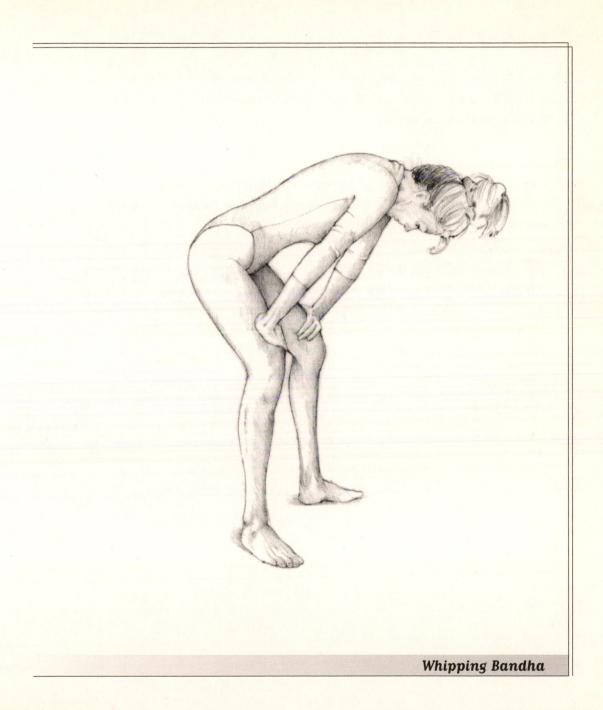

Whipping Bandha

IMPROVE METABOLIC RATE

Vinyasa 7

Slowly increase the pace of this vinyasa as you progress. Start the first repetition slowly; build up speed as you progress to the last repetition, so that you finish a little sweaty and out of breath.

Benefits

Strengthens the lower back and upper body; improves balance; stretches and tones all the muscles of the legs, arms, back, and abdomen; increases overall lean body mass to increase metabolic rate

Focus

Breathe normally but more deeply and vigorously than usual throughout the sequence to increase your body temperature, rid your lungs of stale air, and increase oxygen levels to your blood (and raise your metabolic rate).

Warning: If you have a serious weight problem or suffer from lower-back pain, check with your medical practitioner before attempting this vinyasa.

1. Stand with your feet hip-width apart and your arms hanging at your sides.

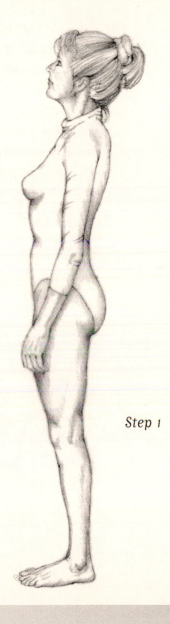

Step 1

Vinyasa 7

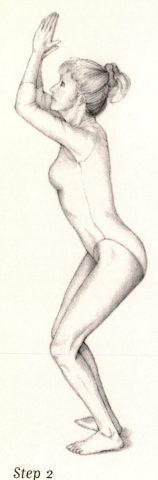

2. Bend your knees and squat, extending both arms out in front of you, then up overhead, with palms parallel to each other and about 12 inches apart. Extend your fingers strongly. Squat deeply, as if you were sitting in a chair, and feel the stretch in your calf muscles.

3. Return to a standing position. Bend forward, and place your palms flat on the floor (bend your knees if necessary).

Step 2

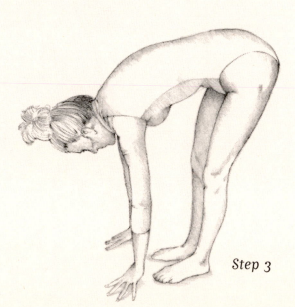

Step 3

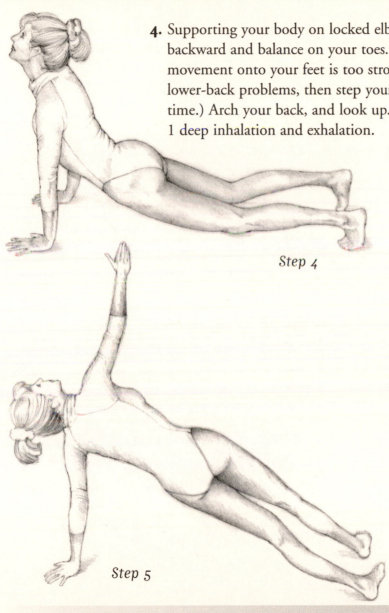

4. Supporting your body on locked elbows, jump both feet backward and balance on your toes. (**Note:** If this jumping movement onto your feet is too strong, or if you have lower-back problems, then step your feet back one at a time.) Arch your back, and look up. Hold the pose for 1 deep inhalation and exhalation.

Step 4

5. Shift your weight onto your left arm. Turn and twist your body away from the floor, cross your right ankle over the back of your left ankle, and lift your right arm to the ceiling. Look up at your right hand. Keep your left elbow locked, and press the toes of your right foot into the floor to help you balance. Hold the balance for 1 deep inhalation and exhalation.

Step 5

Vinyasa 7

6. Return your right arm to the floor, uncross your ankles, and drop your knees to the floor. Inhaling, round your back as you pull your abdominal muscles back up and under your rib cage strongly.

7. Exhaling, sit back on your heels, arms extended on the floor in front of you.

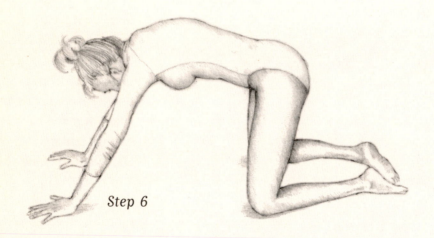

Step 6

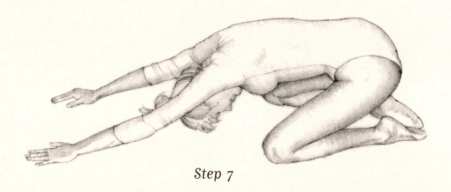

Step 7

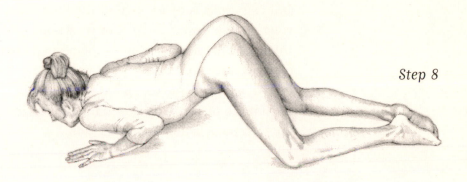

Step 8

8. Inhaling, bend your elbows and slide your chin and chest forward along the floor; keep a strong arch in your lower back.

9. Push your chest through your bent elbows. Exhaling, straighten your arms, drop your hips toward the floor, and arch your body up, with the tops of your feet still on the floor. Support your body on locked elbows, and look up as you take 1 deep inhalation and exhalation.

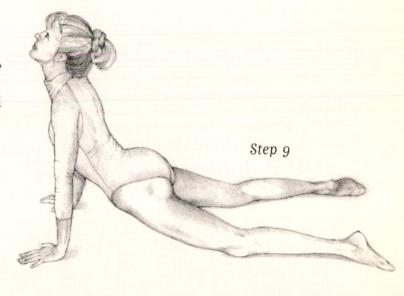

Step 9

Vinyasa 7

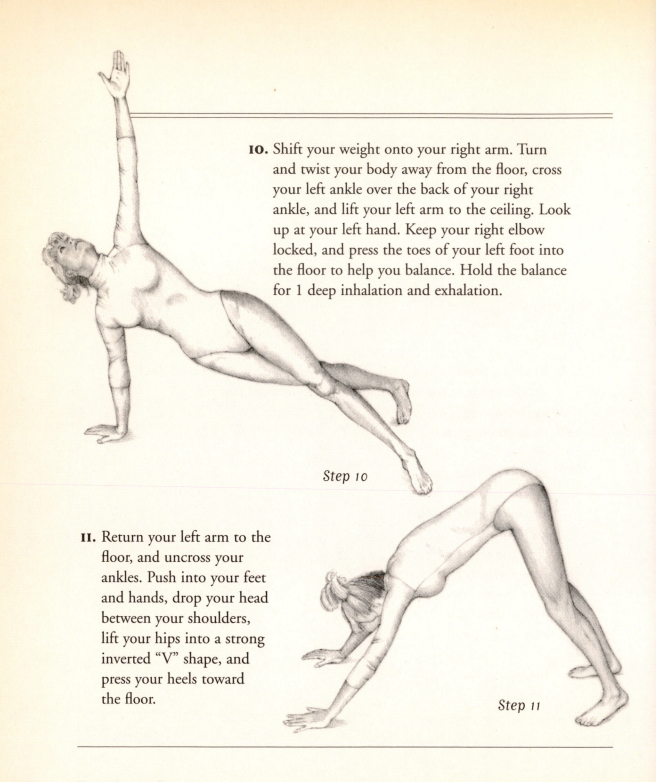

10. Shift your weight onto your right arm. Turn and twist your body away from the floor, cross your left ankle over the back of your right ankle, and lift your left arm to the ceiling. Look up at your left hand. Keep your right elbow locked, and press the toes of your left foot into the floor to help you balance. Hold the balance for 1 deep inhalation and exhalation.

Step 10

11. Return your left arm to the floor, and uncross your ankles. Push into your feet and hands, drop your head between your shoulders, lift your hips into a strong inverted "V" shape, and press your heels toward the floor.

Step 11

12. Inhaling through your nose, extend your right leg up and back, supporting yourself on locked elbows. Lengthen your spine.

13. Exhaling through your mouth forcefully, bend your right knee and bring it to your right elbow. Repeat this extending-and-bending movement 2 more times.

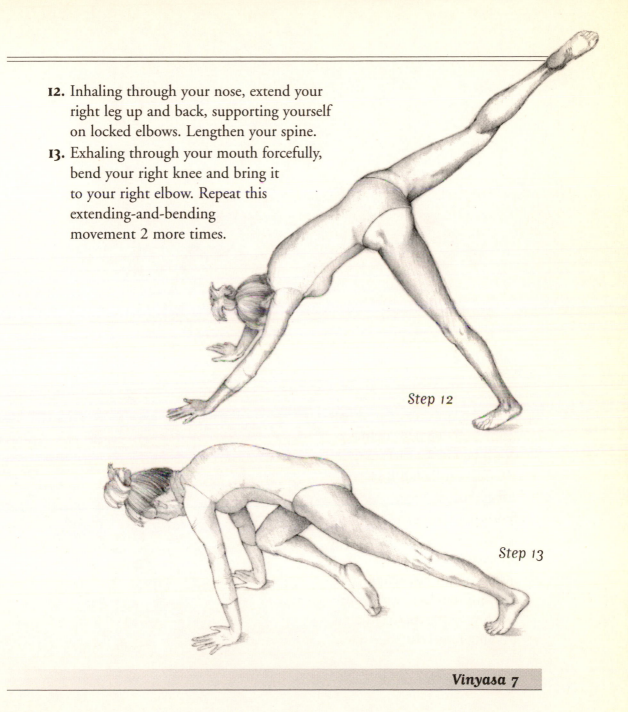

Step 12

Step 13

Vinyasa 7

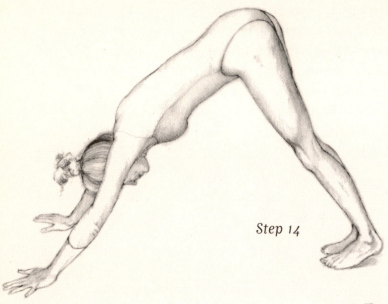

Step 14

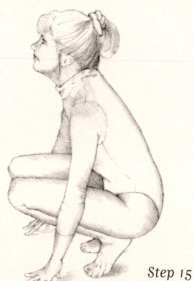

14. After the last extension, exhale while bringing your right leg down beside your left foot. "Walk" your hands back to your feet.

15. Squat for a moment, and take a Full Yoga Breath (see Breathe on page 68 for detailed instructions). Straighten your legs and stand up, with your feet hip-width apart and arms hanging loosely at your sides.

Step 15

16. Repeat the sequence 3 times on the other side, inhaling through your nose when you extend your left leg up and back, and exhaling through the mouth when you bring your bent left leg to your elbow. After the last extension, exhale while bringing your left leg down beside your right foot. "Walk" your hands back to your feet.

17. Repeat the entire sequence (Steps 1–15) for a total of 7 repetitions. Start the first repetition and finish the last repetition using your extended right leg, so you actually will extend the right leg 4 times and the left leg 3 times.

18. Bring your right leg down beside your left foot. "Walk" your hands back to your feet, and return to a standing position.

19. Stand quietly, taking Full Yoga Breaths until your breathing and heart rate have returned to normal. Drink a glass of water to replenish the fluids in your body.

Vinyasa 7

BREATHE

Alternate Nostril Breathing and Right Nostril Breathing

At the 10th International Yoga Therapy Conference, the following breathing sequence was recommended for weight loss: 9 rounds of Alternate Nostril Breathing followed by 27 rounds of Right Nostril Breathing, 3 times per day. This is a very dynamic breathing sequence, so build up to it gently until you are comfortable with the technique.

Warning: If your lungs get tired or if you experience fatigue or irritation, rest and lie down; practice fewer repetitions. Also lie down and rest if your back aches. If your head becomes hot, release the technique and rest for a few moments from the strain.

Alternate Nostril Breathing

Benefits

Brings equal amounts of oxygen to both sides of the brain for effective mental function in both the logical and creative aspects of the mind; improves focus and concentration; calms the nerves; creates mental stillness and focus

Focus

Make your inhalation and exhalation the same length. Feel as if your whole body is centered over the base of your spine, and feel energized as you follow your breath in and out of your nose. Feel the warmth of your breath as you practice.

1. Sit on the floor in Cross-Legged Position, hands resting on your knees. Spine is upright but relaxed. (**Note:** If this position is not comfortable, sit on a folded towel to tilt your hips forward and take the pressure off your knees. Alternatively, sit with your legs stretched out in front, leaning against a wall if necessary, or sit in a chair.)

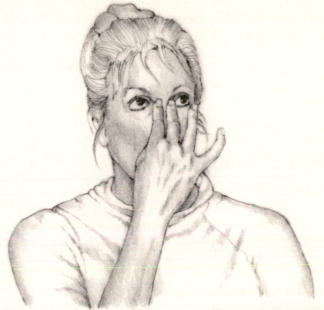

Alternate Nostril Breathing

2. Place the index and middle fingers of your right hand firmly on top of your nose. Rest your right thumb on your cheek next to your right nostril and your right ring finger on your cheek next to your left nostril.

3. Close your right nostril with your thumb, and inhale slowly through your left nostril.

4. Close your left nostril with your ring finger, open your right nostril, and exhale through your right nostril.

5. Inhale through your right nostril, close your right nostril, open your left nostril, and exhale through your left nostril. (Two exhalations—one on each side—complete one round of Alternate Nostril Breathing.)

Alternate Nostril Breathing and Right Nostril Breathing

6. Repeat 8 more rounds. Throughout the day, complete 9 rounds of Alternate Nostril Breathing 2 more times, perhaps after two meals.

(**Note:** If you lose track of your breath, remember this: if you find yourself breathing in, close that nostril, and exhale through your other nostril. If you find yourself breathing out, breathe back in through that same nostril, close it, and exhale through your other nostril.)

Right Nostril Breathing

Benefits
Activates the left hemisphere of the brain, which is associated with active mental abilities; helps to focus concentration and energy

Focus
Pay attention to the movement of your breath in and out of your right nostril and the warmth of the air. Slow the breath down and deepen it as you progress.

1. Sit on the floor in Cross-Legged Position, with your hands resting on your knees. Spine is upright but relaxed. (**Note:** If this position is not comfortable, sit on a folded towel to tilt your hips forward and take the pressure off your knees. Alternatively, sit with your legs stretched out in front, leaning against a wall if necessary, or sit in a chair.)

2. Place the index and middle fingers of your right hand firmly on top of your nose. Rest your right ring finger on your cheek next to your left nostril and your right thumb extended away from your cheek.

3. Close your left nostril; inhale and exhale slowly through your right nostril 27 times. Follow the movement of your breath with concentration.

4. Relax and sit quietly, taking note how you feel. Throughout the day, repeat Right Nostril Breathing 2 more times.

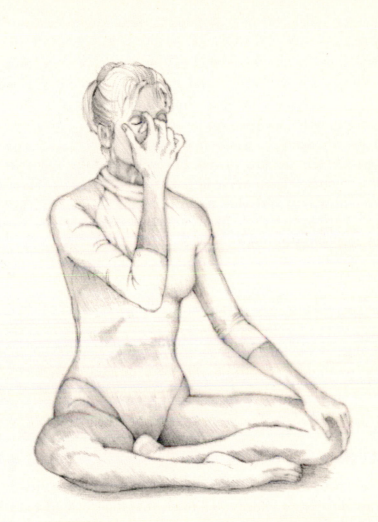

Right Nostril Breathing

Alternate Nostril Breathing and Right Nostril Breathing

VISUALIZE

Release Old Ideas and Limiting Thoughts

Your thoughts can be positive or self-limiting, according to the way that you have colored them with your emotional energy. As you observe your breathing and your mind moves into the rhythm of your breath, your emotions calm down so that you can detach from your emotional self and look objectively at the impact of your thinking on your efforts to reach your goals. The results you receive from this technique will be different each time you try it because the quality of your thoughts changes from day to day.

To survive well in this life, you need to avoid all of the health problems associated with obesity listed in the introduction to this book. Throughout this visualization, mentally assess where you wish to put your energy. You can prevent health problems later on in life by redirecting your energy into positive, healthy, life-sustaining thoughts.

Benefits

Quiets the mind to allow reflection on the quality of thoughts

Focus

Watch the rise and fall of your abdomen or your chest, or concentrate on the warmth of the air coming in through your nose.

(**Note:** If your mind wanders, do not get frustrated; gently draw it back to focus on your breath.)

Cross-Legged Position

1. Sit on the floor in Cross-Legged Position. (**Note:** If this position is not comfortable, sit on a folded towel to tilt your hips forward and take the pressure off your knees. Alternatively, sit with your legs stretched out in front, leaning against a wall if necessary, or sit in a chair.) Rest your hands loosely over your knees, and arch your back a little. Relax your shoulders. Gently drop your chin to your chest.

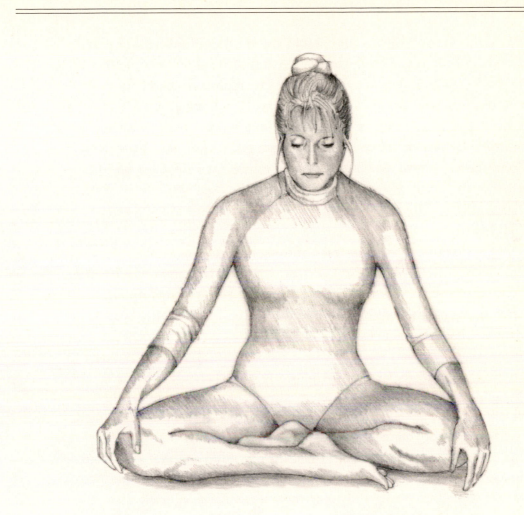

Cross-Legged Position

Release Old Ideas and Limiting Thoughts

2. Watch the rise and fall of your chest as you inhale and exhale. See your abdomen softly round on the inhalation and contract on the exhalation.

3. As you inhale, imagine that you are drawing in positive energy for your relationships, your self-growth, and your goals and aspirations.

4. As you exhale, imagine that you are breathing out any negative energy in your life: feelings of disappointment, anger, resentment, fear, or anxiety.

5. Continue to observe your breath. As you inhale, mentally hang on to the positives in your life; as you exhale, let go of the negatives.

6. Repeat this exercise for 20 breaths as you slow your breathing down slightly.

7. Relax, and return to your natural breathing pattern.

8. Close your eyes. Become as still as a statue so that your mind can be clear, like a pristine lake, with not a ripple to disturb your peace of mind.

9. Let your logical thinking subside and the chatter in your mind become quiet, so that your mind can rest.

10. In the silence, become aware of where you are putting your energy each day. Ask yourself whether you are plugging your energy into negative thoughts or positive thoughts. Energy always follows thought, so check which thoughts are uppermost in your mind when it comes to creating a healthy body for yourself.

11. Imagine that you have a conveyor belt in your mind and that all of your thoughts pass in front of you on this conveyor belt. As you become aware of your thoughts coming and going in your mind, ask yourself

   ➤ What thought form is my energy on right at this moment?
   ➤ Is it an empowering thought or a self-limiting thought? (A self-limiting thought may be something like "I need to lose 10 pounds before I will look good.")

12. When you come across a self-limiting thought, ask yourself
    ➤ Is it true? What evidence do I have for this belief?
    ➤ Does this belief belong to me, or has it been passed down to me by someone or something else (e.g., friends or family, the media, or early teachers)?
    ➤ Do I agree with it?
    ➤ Do I want to put my energy into this thought form to make it a reality?

13. If you do not want to put your energy behind the thought, visualize yourself placing the thought on the conveyor belt of your mind, and watch it go out of sight and out of mind. Take a deep breath, and sigh out the negative energy associated with the self-limiting thought.

14. If you want to keep a particular thought so that you can actualize it, mentally place it in the first energy center, or *chakra*, at the base of your spine, and visualize a vibrant red color glowing around it. (**Note:** The purpose of this chakra is to link the individual with the physical world. It is the foundation for evolving and building the personality. It embraces aspects such as energy, self-expression, ambition, consistency, desire for security, and survival of the self and the species.)

15. Continue this process of releasing negative thoughts and retaining positive thoughts as you sit in the silence for 15 minutes.

16. Open your eyes, and stretch your arms and legs.

Release Old Ideas and Limiting Thoughts

chapter eleven

The Yoga Difference

By practicing the yoga techniques in this book, you'll not only gain lean muscle tissue and increase your metabolism (think "fat burning"), but you'll also get back in touch with your body's needs on a deeper level. You'll learn to distinguish between your physiological need for food and your soul's need for nourishment, which should lessen any dependence on food, alcohol, and other stimulants. Learning this art of inner fulfillment is a lifelong commitment and presents many challenges. Regularly practicing these yoga routines will keep you focused on your goals so that you achieve success and have the energy to enjoy your life to the fullest.

In today's fast-paced society, we often expect results now—instant flight bookings, instant sales purchases, and instant pleasure—but when it comes to reaching and maintaining a healthy weight, this does not apply. When a fad diet fails to result in immediate weight loss, you may feel like a failure. But it's the diets that fail, not you. Rather than looking for an answer in the form of a pill, potion, or diet, turn to the practice of yoga.

Losing a dress size along the way is terrific, and it may make you feel great, but remember that your body is just your outer shell. Underneath that shell is a person with needs, desires, goals, and aspirations. The ability to satisfy your soul and create the reality that you desire plays a big role in your health and well-being.

Nature Takes Its Course

It may surprise you to learn that your body already knows how to regulate your weight. Just 30 minutes of daily yoga practice can be enough to get you in shape. But the key to weight management is to take time out of your busy schedule to create the right conditions to heal imbalances in your body, mind, or emotions that may be contributing to a weight problem. The right conditions include:

➤ Exercising sufficiently as you age, to build enough lean muscle to keep your metabolism high;
➤ Eating as nutritiously as you can;
➤ Keeping your stress levels manageable; and
➤ Creating mind-body harmony.

By completing the routines and practicing the breathing and visualization techniques in this book, you are well on your way to creating the right conditions. You now have a wealth of information and new stress-management skills at your fingertips. You can use these skills simply to lose weight, or to go beyond the immediate benefits of your weight loss. You can take these new skills into other areas of your life. Some changes you might notice include:

➤ Improved self-esteem as a result of changing unhealthy behaviors to healthy ones.
➤ More self-discipline and willpower to help you maintain these changes in your long-term behavior.
➤ The ability to de-stress your body, mind, and emotions by sequential stretching and rhythmic breathing.
➤ The ability to think and act with calm self-assurance and ease.

Inner Nourishment

You have now learned from this book how to nourish your physical needs for a healthy body from within, but you also have the skills to go further and explore your mental, emotional, and spiritual needs as well. For, as Godfrey Devereux, author of the *Hatha Yoga: Breath by Breath*, says: "Hatha yoga is a spiritual practice. In practical terms, yoga involves the release of human potential. This means the full power of your body and the full power of your mind become available. The deeper you go into the practice, the more this potential will fulfill itself."

Imagine how you can use that improved concentration, determination, self-discipline, self-confidence, willpower, physical and mental stamina, and inner calm to bring positive changes to other areas of your life. The power of your mind is unlimited. Following the steps in this book is the first of many challenges to keep you moving forward.

We are each responsible for our own well-being. Take the time to explore all of your inner needs and to satisfy them. Look after the inner needs, and the outer needs will take care of themselves, including keeping you at your healthy optimal weight. Do not settle for second best—you deserve to travel first class all the way in this life! Keep growing, because what you are becoming is inwardly beautiful, and what you see what you see when you look in the mirror is just the tip of your true potential. Enjoy the journey.